This book is dedicated to my wonder woman,

my wife Carmela De Vany,

whose energy, love and humour inspire and nourish me

THE new evolution DIET

and lifestyle programme

The Smart Way to Lose Weight, Feel Great and Live Longer

Professor
Arthur De Vany

Vermilion
LONDON

1 3 5 7 9 10 8 6 4 2

Published in 2011 by Vermilion, an imprint of Ebury Publishing
A Random House Group Company

Copyright © Arthur De Vany 2011

Arthur De Vany has asserted his right to be identified as the author of this
work in accordance with the Copyright, Designs and Patents Act 1988

The Random House Group Limited Reg. No. 954009

Addresses for companies within the Random House Group can be found at
www.randomhouse.co.uk

A CIP catalogue record for this book is available from the British Library

The Random House Group Limited supports The Forest Stewardship Council
(FSC), the leading international forest certification organisation. All our titles that
are printed on Greenpeace-approved FSC-certified paper carry the FSC logo. Our
paper procurement policy can be found at www.rbooks.co.uk/environment

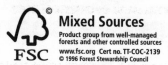

Mixed Sources
Product group from well-managed
forests and other controlled sources
www.fsc.org Cert no. TT-COC-2139
© 1996 Forest Stewardship Council

Designed and set by seagulls.net

Printed in the UK by CPI Mackays, Chatham, ME5 8TD

ISBN 9780091929572

To buy books by your favourite authors and register for offers visit
www.rbooks.co.uk

contents

testimonials

WHAT PEOPLE SAY ABOUT THE NEW EVOLUTION DIET

The New Evolution Diet (NED) has existed for years now, developed by me and adopted by thousands of people who learned about it mostly through my website. I get feedback every day from men and women who follow the diet and exercise plan, and I often learn things even I didn't know – how it works in people's lives and the positive changes it brings about. Even beyond losing weight and getting in shape, adherents tell me the programme has helped with everything from depression and diabetes to acid reflux and haemorrhoids. So I thought I'd begin by sharing some of their stories.

My body is getting strong and my world is lovely again. I have confidence, I am not stressed, I am happy and excited about life … I feel young again, in so many ways. Not only are you changing lives, Art, you are saving them.

At 38 I am stronger, faster, leaner and more alert than I've ever been. Muscle stiffness is virtually a thing of the past, as are hunger and cravings. My 'formal' exercise sessions (as opposed to play) total fifty minutes a week. I couldn't recommend this more.

I'm a 35-year-old female who started this programme at about 146 pounds. I was surprised how easy it was. I dropped 6 pounds in the first week. My skin looked different – bright, tight, and glowing. Without changing anything else, I suddenly had enormous amounts of stamina. And while I've always looked young for my age, I'm now told that I look younger than both my sisters – including one who is 8 years younger than I am.

I am turning 30 this year, and feel orders of magnitude better than I ever have in my life. Thanks to Art De Vany and his protocol I have successfully defeated Seasonal Affective Disorder and acute clinical depression. It really is easy.

Lost 18kg, twenty-year haemorrhoid problem gone, asthma gone, constant cold and chest infections gone, now low body fat rippling with muscle, and flexibility/strength greatly improved (no yoga or stretching), all achieved at middle age with no drugs. Is the happiness I feel the change in hormones or just a natural response to greatly improved health and sense of empowerment? I love the idea that I can be as strong and healthy as I am now in my seventies and beyond. That has to make you feel good! It truly is a new lease on life!

I am shouting it from the rooftops: 'This works – the way the human animal was designed to live!' Thanks from someone enjoying the gift of great physical and mental health restored.

As a personal trainer, I started following the recommendations as a test. Now, two years later, I am much faster and stronger. I don't ever get colds. I never have to worry about being fit. When I tell people I only exercise randomly and for short intervals, they can't believe it. During checkups, the medical staff often ask me if I run marathons and I smile and say, 'No way.'

I have this afternoon returned all insulin syringes to the pharmacy. Now, for the first time in seven years, I no longer require injections. I was at the hospital a week ago and was told to continue to follow the diet with the internist's full support. They concluded, based on blood tests, that my blood sugars are stable, I have no shortage of minerals or vitamins and the complications have disappeared.

I had a reflux problem for a year. It caused hours of coughing at night when the acid trickled up the oesophagus and irritated lesions that the acid had burned in my throat. I was prescribed Zantac, which worked. A year later I switched to this diet and within a day the reflux had disappeared and has not returned – not once – and that's eleven years ago.

I am now 52 years old. At the age of 48, when I found Art De Vany, I was riddled with injuries and had become obese. Now, I am as strong or stronger than I have ever been. I have lost more than eight inches off my waist. I am comfortable, fit, have a better attitude, slower to anger, have more energy, and follow the programme without effort. Further, I just keep getting stronger, thinner and faster. Now my wife has started following the lifestyle. It works, because we're built to live this way.

My doctor told me that I was headed towards pre-diabetes. I discovered Art's blog and read everything on it over a weekend and followed his advice. Within three months I was no longer on blood pressure and cholesterol medication. I went from 18 per cent to 8 per cent body fat, my waist decreased from 35 to 29 inches, and mentally and physically I feel and look better than ever! If it were not for this I would be on some kind of diabetic medication by now. Art, your legacy will live on with my children.

I started a year ago at the age of 54. I haven't been strict with it but it has shown very promising results anyway. My blood pressure has been slightly high for some years. It is now normal. My pulse rate used to be high 70s or early 80s. It was 62 this morning. Art's years of research and rigorous analysis have produced a life-changing and life-saving way of life which mankind can only benefit from. And you never feel hungry or deprived.

Over about a two-month period, I replaced unhealthy foods with these new habits. The results in the subsequent two years have been magic – no more headaches, significantly more energy, muscles appearing and fat melting away. All this with less time spent exercising and more time spent simply having fun biking, skiing and playing. Art is the pre-eminent filter for health information – so far, every one of his suggestions I have implemented has improved my life.

I have learned this much from Art De Vany: your body wants to be healthy and it knows how to be healthy, but our modern practices throw up barriers to health at every turn. Once you begin to incorporate this into your life you will become better able to understand the signals your body sends you. You will crave the food your body needs for health, not the stuff a typical sugar-addicted mind craves. You will find yourself full of energy and gain the discipline needed to exert yourself without exhausting yourself. You will be calm, steady and pleasant in all aspects of life.

I started Art's plan after my daughter was born. A lifetime of chronic migraines and diarrhoea vanished almost immediately and I am now stronger and healthier than I ever have been. This is doubly important because I am 43 years older than my daughter and I am confident that I will be able to raise and guide her well into adulthood in good health and form.

Until I discovered Art's blog, I had a fairly strong body hidden under a fluffy carbohydrate quilt. Thanks to Art, I am leaner, stronger and have never felt or eaten better in my life. Plus, it's so darn easy to stay this way.

introduction
tHe Basis of tHe new evolution Diet

Charles Darwin was overweight and chronically ill. So what can we learn from him about health and fitness?

He teaches us not by example, but by his theory of evolution, which clears away a lot of the nonsense we hear about how to control our weight and get in shape. It also provides us with a powerful model for understanding why we get fat and become weak and chronically ill as we age. Understanding evolution provides us with a path we can take to become healthy and at peace with ourselves.

It's a good place to start, then: What *does* evolution have to do with fitness (or the lack of it)?

This book is based on my decades-long study of weight, diet and health, which has come to be known as Evolutionary Fitness or EF (and has evolved into the New Evolution Diet). It attempts to find guidance in these matters based in part on what life was like roughly 40,000 years ago. This is not out of any nostalgia I have for the

Stone Age, but rather an acknowledgement that, as far as our bodies are concerned, nothing much has changed since then.

So, who were we 40,000 years ago? Our ancestors of that era were tall, muscular and lean. Food was often scarce. Exercise (meaning the physical activity required to survive) was made up of heavy labour plus intense but brief 'fight or flight' emergencies. Our ancestors retained their health throughout their lives, though their years were considerably fewer than ours.

Homo erectus, our ancestor from one million years ago, could go out today and buy a suit (42 long) at Ralph Lauren and walk the streets of New York with little notice. He would be tall and lean, built like a basketball guard. A Cro-Magnon who roamed the earth 40,000 years ago might buy an Armani (44 long) – they had a better sense of style than *Homo erectus*, which is evident in the art objects and cave paintings they left for us to enjoy. Cro-Magnon might look more like a rugby player; he would be taller than most males now and would be lean, muscular and very powerful – a devastating athlete. He would also have a bigger brain than we have. All this can be inferred from their skeletons, from the capabilities of contemporary hunter-gatherers, and through comparisons between other animals living in the laboratory and in the wild.

Similarly, a female Cro-Magnon would be slender, a bit taller than a modern female, and would have the classic hourglass shape and posture of a graceful woman. She might be a supermodel, but not a skinny, starved waif – she'd have a great figure, based on the depictions of shapely women found in their art.

Modern humans carry a copy of the same genes as our Cro-Magnon ancestors from just 40,000 years ago. At least 70 per cent of humans alive today can trace their genes to the small band of Cro-Magnon humans who lived through the last Ice Age. The origins of the seven tribes of humans living in Europe can be traced to seven males who lived between 100,000 and 40,000 BC.

Why, then, does this same genetic material, which once expressed health and muscular leanness in our ancestors, now express obesity and chronic illness? The answer is in the interaction between our genes and their surroundings – in other words, our modern, affluent society.

In short, we are genetically engineered to thrive in a different world. I believe that if you took a prehistoric hunter-gatherer and placed him or her in our environment, he or she would behave just as we do and would eventually suffer the same problems. We know this is true because we *are* hunter-gatherers and we *do* suffer. We also know that when contemporary hunter-gatherers enter industrialised society, they end up with our bad habits and chronic ailments.

This brings us to a key concept to keep in mind as you read on. We stopped evolving and adapting when food was scarce and life was full of arduous physical activity. Hence, our bodies instruct us to eat everything we can lay our hands on and exert ourselves as little as possible.

That's right. We are, in essence, programmed to be lazy overeaters.

This was a perfect strategy for success thousands of years ago, but it is a recipe for disaster today. No human could survive in 40,000 BC unless they ate whenever food was available. They knew that famine was always close at hand. Eat now or you might not survive to eat another day. And take care to expend as little energy as possible, because even then you'll end up exerting yourself a great deal. Burning more calories than absolutely necessary was a threat to survival.

In the modern world, a hunter-gatherer would follow those same principles: he'd eat a lot and move little. And he would suffer all the ills we do, now that the situation has been turned upside down, and food is abundant while physical activity has become more or less voluntary. This explains why most diet and exercise advice is pointless. To move more and eat less is a direct contradiction of our genetically engineered impulses.

Our forager ancestors would seek high-energy (meaning high-calorie, high-fat) foods that could be obtained at the lowest energy cost. They would eat or not depending on what they could find or kill, meaning mealtime was a fairly unpredictable thing. They would move when hungry (or when being pursued) and relax once fed – like wild animals do today. Their movements would be sporadic, meaning short periods of intense activity (hunting, hauling, climbing, running) separated by long stretches of languid rest and play. There would be unpredictable intervals of low food intake, even occasional starvation, interwoven with times of abundance. This is the environment for which our behaviour and our metabolism are designed. As far as our genes are concerned, this is still the way of the world. Only we know different.

*

Why *do* we get fat and sick? They are odd questions from an evolutionary perspective, because ancestral humans were not overweight. Nor were they ill in the ways we become in our civilised world today. We began getting fat and suffering new diseases once we ceased to live as hunter-gatherers and instead became farmers.

Now we suffer from a host of chronic 'Western' diseases that were virtually unknown among our early ancestors and are largely absent even among contemporary hunter-gatherers living in traditional ways. The list is long and depressingly familiar: obesity, adult-onset diabetes, hypertension, cardiovascular disease, Alzheimer's, and so on.

Each of these modern ailments is recognised to be a sickness of metabolism and inflammation. Something in modern life is disturbing the internal systems that evolution handed down to us.

In general, our bodies do not seem to thrive on modern life, where inactivity is imposed by work and where alcohol, drugs (prescription and otherwise) and even food are abused. Nor do our minds seem to enjoy contemporary living. Humans today probably experience more chronic stress than our ancestors did, whose stresses would have been acute and episodic. The 'fight or flight' instincts our ancestors relied upon to escape danger are triggered today in innumerable ways, but without resolution. The resulting chronic stress is a potent source of misery and disease. Even our wealth and possessions do not bring satisfaction, because our minds evolved at a time when such things were meaningless.

You can see the evolutionary history of our species in the development of the human foetus. The child in gestation looks like a minnow at first, then like a tadpole, then a frog or maybe a large shrimp. Little buds poke out where limbs develop; the ribs of the fishlike skeleton fuse to form a pelvis; the head enlarges and eye buds pop out and the foetus starts to resemble a pale, curled-up dolphin. Only gradually does it develop into something that looks human.

A human baby born today would just as easily thrive 40,000 years ago. And a baby born in 40,000 BC would look just like a baby born today. They would have the same genes and develop into normal babies and adults in either era. Each child born today carries genes that prepare it for the life of a hunter-gatherer, the occupation of every human who has ever lived except for we few generations who came after the recent invention of agriculture 10,000 years ago.

The remarkable thing is that we do so well in the modern world. That little baby born today has no more genetic instructions on how to live and survive now than the one born 40,000 years ago. Today's baby is no stronger, smarter or better suited for life than one born in the distant past. Even though the Palaeolithic child grew up to make stone chips and spears and to hunt mammoth, it uses the same brain modules and learning skills that let the modern one grow up to make computer chips and business deals and to hunt for theorems in an abstract mathematical space.

This is astonishing but true. How does that child who is wired to be a hunter-gatherer learn to be a nuclear physicist? Or a politician? It doesn't seem possible. But they have the same brain and the same body and can therefore have the same thoughts, and with enough training can do the same things. They are different only because they live in different worlds, and there is the rub.

That baby whose genes, brain and body expect it to be a forager grows up to be a sales manager or a tax account-ant. Instead of roaming the African savannah scrounging for food, she shops on the highstreet or at the supermar-ket. Rather than pursuing antelope, he tracks financial flows on a spreadsheet. None of our ancestors ever craved a French fry or drank a sugary soft drink.

Many of the foods we eat today are completely novel substances from an evolutionary perspective. We do know that our predecessors were incomparably better nourished than we are, and that they were very powerful, fit and not fat. Their activity levels are more typical of elite athletes than office workers.

An evolutionary adaptation is a capability or trait that confers a particular advantage in a specific environment. If modern circumstances differ from the ones to which we were adapted, then our genes may actually be disadvantageous today. As I mentioned, our brains are hard-wired for a 'fight or flight' response to danger and stressful situations. But modern life presents us with many such moments that we can neither fight nor flee from. You can't punch your boss in the nose, or run away from an overdue mortgage payment. We're not built to handle those stresses well, and in fact we don't.

Here's another example: the human preference for sweet tastes and fat was developed in an environment where such treats were rare and signalled dense, useful energy. This once-helpful adaptation is the downfall of many a dieter today. It's what makes it hard to resist fats and sweets, especially when they are all around us.

Even with all that, life today is better than ever. It is safer, and we are all but free of the many pathogens and parasites that threatened our ancestors. Far fewer infants die now than did in the Palaeolithic era. Life expectancy is higher not only at birth, but also at all ages now.

Our ancestors had a higher probability of death at every age than we do, but they lived a smaller portion of their lives in disability. Modern humans live longer but age more rapidly than our prehistoric ancestors, and we live more of our lives in chronic illness. (This, arguably, is better than not living at all.) Our forebears were fit well into their advanced years. A good deal of what we call 'normal ageing' is a modern condition that is more akin to disease than any natural state of growing older.

There is a reason for this. Using the scientific jargon, we are active genotypes trying to live as sedentary phenotypes. In plain English, that means we are not living as we were built to live. Our genes were forged in an environment where activity was mandatory – you were active or you starved or were eaten. This created strong selective pressure for genes encoding a smart, physically adept individual capable of very high activity levels. Humans are among the most active of species, and we carry energetically expensive brains to boot. Our energy expenditures rank high among all animals – or should I say they once did.

The sedentary phenotype, *Homo sedentarius*, is the typical modern citizen who gets no exercise, becomes obese, unfit, chronically ill, and ages rapidly. He ignores his biological need for activity. Inactivity and obesity alter the expression of your genes, and this is what produces the whole modern array of chronic, debilitating ailments.

So, regular exercise is not just something you do to improve your health and drop a little fat. It is not an 'intervention', as some health professionals call it. It is absolutely essential to a healthy life – as necessary as food, water and air. You exercise because the length and quality of your life depend upon it.

What happens to astronauts is pretty convincing evidence of the necessity of activity. The space traveller's body wastes away when it is in a zero-gravity environment. They must exercise or they will not last to the end of the mission. Even when they do work out, they return to earth having lost a good deal of their muscle, organ, heart and skeletal tissue (and probably brain tissue, too).

A couch astronaut does no less damage. It just takes longer for him to waste away because gravity is still pulling on him and he has to get up now and then. The lean body mass of the couch astronaut wastes away even as he grows in circumference, total body mass and percentage body fat. This altered body composition will age him rapidly because he is also losing his metabolic fitness.

The good news in all this is that our genes are not the sum total of our destiny; we can alter our gene expression for better or worse.

One thing we can do in that regard is to eat properly. A forager moving over the savannah in the quest for food will encounter patches of edible plants in great variety and in seasonal abundance (even in the marginal environments that contemporary hunter-gatherers occupy, there may be 300 edible plants). Foraging for animal sources offers its own rewards. One big kill may equal thousands of plants in energy, and will contain more protein and valuable fatty acids as well. We are adapted to consume a large and changing variety of foods. It is known that people who consume a varied diet experience superior health and longevity compared to those who eat from a monotonous palette.

As with food, variety in activity is healthy. The lack of it leads to overwork and not enough play or rest. I believe we should model our activities on the movements of children at play or predators at work. This leads to a rather radical but peaceful departure from a good deal of common advice regarding exercise.

I take life easier than almost anyone I know, but when I exercise I do it as though my life depends upon it (which it does). I never work out for more than an hour and a half per week, and I sometimes go days without exercising at all. I spend more time doing nothing than most people I know – really nothing, not reading or watching television, just roaming the hills near our home, or taking easy walks with my wife, or lying on the grass with my dogs and watching the sky. I even organise my work life that way, mixing intensely productive periods with stretches of pure laziness.

A forager may spend many fruitless hours in the search for high-energy animal foods, subsisting on plants until the next kill. I think human metabolism is adapted to this pattern of intermittent variety in food sources and periodic fasting mixed with varying activity levels. The chronic routine of three balanced meals a day and two snacks combined with the chronic routine of repetitive exercise just does not square with how our metabolism is built to function. There must be a periodic emptying of energy reserves through activity and intermittent hunger. Unless we do this, I don't think it is possible to overcome the instinct to eat more calories than we burn that allowed our hunter-gatherer ancestors to survive and pass their genes on to us.

A large body of genetic research supports this view, as I will discuss in various places throughout the book. The same research supports the view that it is the carbohydrate in our diets that hinders our metabolism from functioning as evolution intended.

Darwin put it this way: 'Reproduction is how life commutes its death sentence.' What that means is that our DNA has to decide whether to repair itself or to depend on our sexual reproduction to carry our genes forward. During times of plenty, our DNA allows us to reproduce. When resources are scarce, it focuses on self-repair, which extends our good health and longevity. DNA takes its signal from carbohydrate – if it exists in abundance, our DNA assumes that food is plentiful, and so it can rely on our reproduction impulses. That mechanism is a powerful reason for restricting our carb intake – doing so triggers our self-repair processes. It also helps us to control our weight.

The strategies that come from the evolutionary perspective are simple and powerful. Here are the guiding principles:

1   Enjoy the pleasure of food and do not count or restrict calories. Eat a diet low in glucose and starch that is similar (but not identical) to the one humans lived with for thousands of years as human metabolism evolved.

2   Do not starve yourself, but *do* go hungry episodically, for brief periods. That just means you should practise partial fasting once a week or so. An easy way to do that is to skip meals when you have other things to do.

3 Exercise less, not more, but with more playfulness and intensity. Exercise for the pleasure of the sensations, not to burn calories. Exercise to create a beautiful, strong body with a high resting metabolism and a large physiological capacity to move through life easily and handle stress and challenges easily.

By giving up on the unsuccessful 'eat less, exercise more' approach to health, you will suffer far less stress. By varying your eating patterns, the foods you eat and your activity, you will transform your chronic, debilitating stress into episodes of brief, energising, acute stress that are beneficial.

By exercising more like a wild animal than a robot, you will build a physical capacity that brings a kind of fearless-ness and a sense of confidence that you are up to any situation you may face. More intense but brief exercise supplies energy to the brain to offset hunger in a way that long and slow exercise cannot.

Muscle is medicine; it releases many substances that promote health. Fat is poison; it sends forth chemicals that disrupt metabolism and promote chronic disease and ageing. Building muscle alters metabolism to direct energy and nutrients to our brain and muscle and deny them to fat. By becoming slender and muscular we can reach a balance of fat and muscle that makes it easy to maintain weight in a stable range.

There is no need for willpower on this diet because you do not restrict calories. Eating well will lead your metabolism to adjust itself and send all your energy to your brain and muscle and not to your fat stores. When the ratio of muscle to fat – your body composition – reaches a healthy point, everything else falls into place. Believe me, you do *not* want to lose weight; you want to achieve a healthy balance of muscle and fat. The number on the scale is meaningless.

If it sounds easy, that's because it *is*. Please allow me to show you.

one
Before you Begin: eight things to measure

Every diet and exercise plan tells you to consult with your doctor before you start, and this one is no different. But I also suggest that you make sure to measure some things your physician might not automatically check. Some of these items are part of a standard annual checkup, but others are not. A few are simply to determine just how much room for improvement you have; you might want to check them now, and then six months from now, to measure your progress. All are important to health and longevity. I depend on these benchmarks myself to tell me how I'm doing.

1. INSULIN

This may be the single most important thing you can test. Your fasting insulin level is an indicator of your overall metabolic health, plain and simple. Insulin is so central to metabolism that it can accurately predict the outcomes of other tests that are commonly done. Excessive insulin is associated with other worrisome values, such as high triglycerides and high blood pressure; low good (HDL) cholesterol, high bad (LDL) cholesterol, high C-reactive protein (from inflammation); and elevated leptin (leptin and insulin work together, so when both are high obesity is often present). Lastly, your insulin levels will tell you something of your internal fat deposits. A person who has a big waistline and high insulin probably has metabolic damage.

Among contemporary hunter-gatherers, fasting insulin is 5. Mine is at the lowest level the lab is able to measure – 2.0 (for a full list of how I measure up to these benchmarks, see the table at the end of this chapter). Diabetics have fasting insulin levels in a range of 13.5 to 17.6. I have known diabetics whose fasting insulin was above 40. Average fasting insulin is 11.4 in a national American study of 3,000 people, which is still far too high. Physicians typically will not measure insulin levels unless they suspect a problem, so you may need to ask yours to prescribe this blood test for you.

2. OBESITY OR BODY COMPOSITION

Because fat can be thought of as an organ that secretes numerous harmful hormones, you really want to know how much of it you carry. Fat also intrudes into other organs and tissues, disturbing their function. Fat is the primary site of inflammation; as fat cells die they release their contents, and the immune system floods in to soak up the debris, causing inflammation.

In addition to knowing how much fat you carry, it's important to consider how much of it is deep visceral fat and how much is subcutaneous, meaning the kind right under the skin. It is the deep fat that causes most of the damage.

Body composition can be measured accurately using the impedance or immersion methods, which give a reliable approximation of total fat. The caliper method is even more commonly used, but is less accurate; fat has to be measured at seven to twelve sites on the body for precision, and not many people want to go through all that trouble. Short of computer imaging, there is no way to tell precisely how much of each type of fat you have. There are home scales that measure weight, body fat and a variety of other things, but in my experience they are not terribly accurate.

Simply looking at yourself in a mirror reveals a great deal – all you need to know in fact. One should have the X-look, male or female. That means the waist-to-hip ratio ought to be about 0.8 for a male and 0.7 for a female (meaning a man's waist ought to be 80 per cent of the size of his hips; a woman's, 70 per cent). You know when that ratio looks right. Deep visceral fat pushes the gut out at the belly button. Someone with excessive visceral fat will have a somewhat robust look because the fat doesn't sag, and his face will have some colour to it. The colour isn't ruddy good health, it's a sign of inflammation; the face will also be puffy. He or she will look somewhat husky because metabolic syndrome causes fats and glycogen, a form of sugar, to build up in muscles, giving them a bigger look. Since he or she spends a lot of time sitting, an activity that promotes poor metabolism, someone with metabolic syndrome will have reduced muscle mass in the buttocks and legs – their trousers will just hang.

Doctors say that apple-shaped obesity – where the fat is concentrated around the mid-section – indicates a strong likelihood of cardiac disease. A waistline of over 40 inches in men and 35 in women can be taken as a warning sign of impending heart trouble. So you can start your measuring there.

Someone with excessive subcutaneous fat will have fat that hangs over the belt, or will have the familiar 'muffin top' when squeezed into jeans. He or she will also have fat arms, hips and thighs. This pear-shaped body is somewhat less prone to the metabolic syndrome, but all obesity causes problems.

Most doctors will weigh you, and then perhaps compute your body mass index (BMI – your weight in kilograms divided by your height in metres squared). But you can have a 'healthy' BMI according to the charts and still be too fat for optimum health. For example, you may have low weight due to not enough muscle tissue but still have too much fat. Such skinny-fat individuals look thin and may not be overweight according to the charts. But with such poor body composition, that person is at risk of diabetes. Older individuals tend to lose muscle and replace it with fat, meaning they are at risk even if the BMI number says otherwise. They may also lose weight from osteoporosis while becoming fatter.

Conversely, a lean, muscular person may have a high BMI. I am six-foot-one and weigh 14 stone – my BMI is therefore 26.4. According to the standard I am slightly overweight, a silly conclusion when you consider that my body fat is less than 8 per cent. Muscle weighs more than fat, and most athletes fall into the overweight category by the BMI standard.

For the non-athletic population, BMI is a reasonable measure and predictor of metabolic syndrome and the diseases it causes. The chances of death from cancer rise with BMI and so do the risks of many other diseases. The risk of death from cancer actually doubles from the leanest group to the fattest.

3. STRENGTH

Strength is a reliable predictor of mortality. The stronger you are, the less likely you are to die soon. You are also less likely to get cancer, diabetes, heart disease, to have elevated triglycerides, insulin resistance, low HDL, high C-reactive protein (CRP – see later on in this chapter), or to become obese.

A person's life expectancy is a stair-step function of their strength; the strongest survive longer than the next strongest, and so on down the line. When testing is done and people are ranked according to strength, those in the top quarter live longer than those in the quarter below, and they live even longer than those in each of the lower quarters.

How strong should you be? As strong as you can get, because muscle is medicine against developing metabolic diseases. In effect, strength is a measure of your lean muscle mass, the primary site where your body disposes of glucose. Muscle is also your engine for life. The stronger you are, the more active you will be simply because you expend less effort in everything you do. It may take all the power a weak person has to climb a flight of stairs that a strong person can ascend effortlessly.

Strength may be tested in various ways; for example, grip strength is often used because it is convenient. There is a gripper device that some trainers and others use to measure this. But it is less reliable than a test that involves a large muscle group, such as the legs or back. The leg press is reliable because it involves many muscle groups and a large portion of the body's lean muscle mass. If, using two legs, you are able to press twice your body weight, you are in the elite group. Cancer researcher Jonathan R. Ruiz and his co-authors tested more than 8,000 subjects aged from 20 to 80 for muscular strength. They grouped individuals into three categories of strength and found that the age-adjusted risk of cancer was 17.5 per thousand in the weakest group, 11.0 in the middle group, and 10.3 in the strongest group. The weaker groups also had higher blood pressure, higher cholesterol, more cardiovascular disease and greater incidence of diabetes.

4. PHYSIOLOGICAL CAPACITY

Power is strength in action – the combination of speed and strength. Since we know that inflammation kills the valuable fast-twitch muscle fibres, we want to see how much of this precious resource we have available. Physiological capacity – physical power – is a measure of your metabolic headroom, the space where your life occurs.

There are no standard tests for capacity, but more is always better. Thinking of physiological capacity as your fight or flight capability suggests at least one good way to measure this. Football and rugby players are tested in the fifty or hundred metre dash. Your time in either one is a good measure of your ability to respond to a flight challenge. You can chart your progress accurately if you time your fifty metre dash once a month. You may at first have to walk the distance, then run it easily, then sprint lightly, building to a harder run as you progress. Of all athletes, those who sprint – basketball players, soccer players, certain positions in American football – are the most capable and have the best bodies.

Joggers are poor sprinters and often have terrible bodies. Jogging is a useless exercise, as I explain later in this book. For now, suffice it to say that no caveman ever jogged while pursuing dinner or being chased by a predator. You either sprinted or you starved, or were dinner yourself.

If you are so far gone that you hesitate to sprint, you have powerful evidence that your physiological capacity is lousy. It seems that adults are reluctant to sprint and so they lose the great benefits of this most important capacity. There is no good reason to lose this talent; it expresses our inner animal. It is a great mood lifter. Try it. Sprinting on a stationary bicycle is safer and easier to do than running in a field.

I also suggest measuring physiological capacity based on METs (metabolic equivalent of task). A MET is measured as a multiple of your resting metabolic rate, so a reading of 5 METs means you generated 5 times your resting metabolic rate. Children at play generate around 10 METs of peak power. The previously mentioned Ruiz study found that the maximal METs were 11.5 in the lowest strength category, 12.5 in the middle and 13.4 in the upper category. Some cardio machines measure METs. I don't recommend doing much cardio exercise, at least as it is usually defined, but use one of these machines occasionally just to measure your capability.

5. TESTOSTERONE

This is an important hormone for males and females. Testosterone controls body composition for both sexes and is important for vitality. Low testosterone is associated with poor body composition, bad mood, depression, high blood pressure, low strength and energy, and metabolic syndrome. It could be used as a leading indicator of ageing since it begins to decline in most males right after full growth is attained. Over-training and stress cause low testosterone. Marathon runners have *very* low testosterone, and so do some bodybuilders who over-train.

There are no known supplements that will raise testosterone because the level is tightly controlled in the body, but these suggestions may help:

* Cut the booze
* Drop the sugar
* Do high-intensity exercise
* Eat celery, because it raises testosterone level
* Men, run cool water over your testicles after a shower

6. C-REACTIVE PROTEIN (CRP)

This is among the most reliable predictors of cardiovascular inflammation and heart disease. As a result, most doctors will now test for it. The research strongly supports the view that heart disease is a disease of inflammation, which is itself a by-product of obesity. CRP predicts cardiac events more accurately than levels of triglycerides, cholesterol or the ratio of either triglycerides or LDL cholesterol to HDL. Obesity greatly elevates CRP because when the body has a large number of fat cells, the intrinsic rate of fat-cell death increases – a fat person will have about three times as many fat-cell deaths as a lean person. A dying fat cell prompts the immune system to clean up the debris; this means that an overweight person's immune system is being taxed more than that of someone weighing less. And inflammation also damages healthy tissues, such as the vascular lining.

The healthy reference range for CRP is 0 to 2.13. My CRP test comes back negative, but with no number. I would guess that my reading is near the lower limit. This is a consequence of the low inflammatory burden of my diet and my low body fat. I suspect it is also from my intake of antioxidants in my diet and in my supplements (which I will discuss later in this book).

7. GOOD AND BAD CHOLESTEROL

HDL (high-density lipoprotein) is the so-called 'good' cholesterol. It gets its name from its ability to transport lipids back to the liver where they can be metabolised. HDL inhibits inflammation by inhibiting TNA-alpha, an important inflammatory and gene expression activator. LDL (very low-density lipoprotein) is the 'bad' cholesterol, the most readily oxidised form that forms lesions in the blood vessels when it becomes oxidised and engulfed by macrophages of the immune system.

When I enter my values in the WolframAlpha science search engine for heart disease, the formula (based on NHANES data) gives my ten-year risk of heart disease at 2.7 per cent. My wife's readings are similar to mine but they were not so good until she began to eat the way I do. We are going to be happily married for a long time in spite of our age.

8. TRIGLYCERIDES

Simply put, triglycerides are fats circulating in the bloodstream. Elevated triglycerides are almost always the result of metabolic disease. When insulin is chronically high and insulin resistance sets in, the body metabolises glucose. Meanwhile, the fats just sit there in the bloodstream, to be oxidised by the free radicals. This is where the real problem is. Your doctor should also measure the ratio of triglycerides to good cholesterol. That's because, after CRP, the ratio of triglycerides to good cholesterol is the best predictor of cardiovascular disease. You can discuss the reference range with your doctor to assess your risk.

As I said at the start, most of these measures must be ordered by a physician and carried out in the lab, but they are worth the effort and the extra expense.

MY BENCHMARK LEVELS

	My level	Comment
Insulin	2.0	average insulin levels are around 11.4
BMI	26.4	BMI can be misleading if you have a lot of muscle
Strength Leg press	400lb +	using just one leg!
Physiological capacity 40-yard dash	5 seconds	
Maximal METS	30	more than twice the upper-strength level (in the Ruiz study)
Testosterone	660	normal for 20- and 30-year-olds
C-reactive protein	negative	healthy is between 0 and 2.13

	My level	Comment
Cholesterol		
HDL (good)	2.4	1.0 is common in mild diabetics
LDL (bad)	0.3	2.7 is common in mild diabetics
Triglycerides	0.5	near the bottom of the range
Triglycerides:		
T/HDL ratio	0.2	in the zero-risk range

two
tHe new evolution Diet

You want to eat smart. I want you to eat smart. So what would a smart diet look like?

It would reduce the amount of energy (meaning food) you feel like consuming at the same time that it increases the amount of energy you feel like spending. And this would occur spontaneously, without any thoughts of cutting calories or exercising more or anything else. It would just happen.

A smart diet would improve the quality of your life by giving you more energy to expend on work, family and play. It would please the palate with beautiful food that is completely nutritious. It would eliminate anything that interferes with your metabolism or sets off your immune system. A smart diet should rely on the millions of years of evolutionary design built into your appetite and metabolism to solve the problem of managing energy naturally, without a conscious plan.

The New Evolution Diet is a smart diet. It is relaxed because it does not restrict calories – you eat all you want from a wide selection of fresh and nutritious foods that are delicious, aesthetically pleasing and satisfying. It is not a 'top down' menu where you must follow directions and rigidly adhere to a schedule of meals and snacks or restrict your calories. There are no rules. Rules are self-defeating because nobody wants to be told what to eat or do – 'That's why I became an adult,' to borrow a line from Bob Newhart. A command-and-control diet creates stress. Stress causes the release of cortisol, a hormone that promotes insulin resistance. So, stressing over diet and exercise is self-defeating – it actually makes you fatter.

It may be impossible to overeat on this diet because it is so complete and filling – it supplies the brain with all the energy and nutrients it needs while promoting a sensation of fullness in the stomach. That brain–stomach connection is important. When your brain is well nourished, your mind will forget about food. When it is improperly nourished, your brain becomes anxious and selfish and can think only about the next feeding. Then you become lazy because your brain curtails physical activity in order to protect its own energy supply. That means your body stops burning fat.

I want to emphasise this: a well-fed brain reduces your appetite and makes moving your body a pleasure. But when your brain is improperly nourished, it orders you to keep on eating.

Can you see how this dispels the hopelessly simple and damning explanation that is usually given for obesity? You are not overweight because you eat too much and move too little. You eat too much and expend too little energy because you are overweight. Put another way, you are not *what* you eat; you are what your metabolism *does* with what you eat.

So, we have to eat the right foods and avoid the wrong ones in order to keep brain and body supplied with energy. Evolution designed your metabolism to perform that job, so long as you eat properly. Your metabolism wants you to have the only thing that matters: proper body composition, meaning the correct balance of muscle and fat. It doesn't care how many pounds you weigh. Believe it or not, that number will soon be irrelevant to you, too. It will become effortless for you to have a lean, beautiful, active body and a healthy, energetic brain.

Many fad diets will encourage snacking throughout the course of the day. I think this is done to keep from scaring dieters away, but it's not a good idea. You should be eating enough in your regular meals to keep you satisfied. If you're not, adjust that rather than adding three daily mini-meals. The biggest problem with snacks is this: every time you eat, you turn off your body's fat-burning mechanism. That's because your metabolism will always burn glucose before fat, and snacks usually contain at least some glucose. So, snacking actually thwarts your efforts to control weight. Eating between meals also keeps your insulin level higher than it needs to be.

I do sometimes snack, but only under certain circumstances. If I'm going to miss a meal, I will have a snack instead, maybe a slice of turkey breast. Or, before a meal, I may have a handful of nuts, some celery or a pear – just to begin filling my belly and cutting my appetite.

In the early days of the diet, you may feel the need for an occasional snack. You should have one if absolutely necessary, but make it fruit, vegetables, nuts or lean meat – no carbs. Remember that if you just persevere and give your metabolism a chance to adjust to the new eating regime you've adopted, you won't need to snack. And you'll be better off as a result.

In the final analysis, the quality of your life should determine how much you eat. Instead of obsessing over how much you take in and then trying to burn it all off, you should focus on living a high-quality life and then eat to fulfil your energy demand. The pleasure and quality of life comes from the energy you spend.

So, what are you supposed to eat? In a later chapter, I have explained my eating habits as a way of suggesting some you might adopt. I am going to assume that you're not the kind of person who needs someone to dictate exactly what you will eat every day for the rest of your life. Here, as briefly as I can manage, is the New Evolution Diet.

*

In the United States, nutritional authorities created and then refined, over the years, the familiar food pyramid: the grouping of all foods into categories of varying sizes in order to illustrate how much of each you should eat.

My diet totally eliminates two of the five categories – grain-based foods and dairy – because they are harmful and shouldn't be eaten at all. And since beans, legumes and seeds are not so great for you, they should be cut, if not eliminated.

One rationale for banishing grain-based foods – that is, anything made with flour of any kind, or derived from corn or other grains – is that these did not exist when our genes stopped evolving, and so our bodies are not equipped to metabolise them. That is true, but there's an even better and more practical reason: Simple carbohydrates and sugar have almost single-handedly caused our current plagues of obesity and type-2 diabetes. That includes bread, pasta and anything else baked. Rice, too, is a grain to be avoided.

Having said all that, I should add that I sometimes break the above commandment. I happen to love tacos, which contain both simple carbs *and* fats. I fill them with healthy ingredients, such as fish and vegetables, but the fact remains that 40,000 years ago, nobody ate tacos. However, the occasional deviation from the norm is fine – our goal is not to replicate exactly the Palaeo diet, just to learn from it. So I don't overdo it with tacos or other such treats, such as my favourite dessert, which is cheesecake. But I take occasional pleasure from them all the same.

You've been led to believe that beans and legumes are healthy, I know, but in fact they are a mixed blessing. They contain plant proteins and other substances that cause a wide variety of ills, which more than wipe out whatever benefits they may confer. Some even contain toxins. I realise that telling you to stay away from beans is practically heresy, but I'll explain my reasons in more detail later in this chapter.

To replace the old food pyramid, I devised one of my own. The shape conveys the general idea, but it cannot show the variation in food sources, which is a very important consideration. The water is a bit out of proportion because you should not force yourself to drink. Simply rely on your thirst to indicate your needs. Over-hydration is not healthy and can even, in extreme cases, be fatal. Leave the water bottle at home.

THE NEW EVOLUTION DIET FOOD PYRAMID

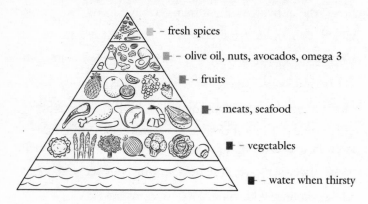

- – fresh spices

- – olive oil, nuts, avocados, omega 3

- – fruits

- – meats, seafood

- – vegetables

- – water when thirsty

NEW EVOLUTION DIET – BASIC GUIDELINES

* Eat whole foods. These would be foods that you (or someone else) can either pick or catch and kill.
* Eat at least some food raw. Have a salad or something uncooked once a day.
* Eat a wide variety of foods. This allows you to receive a larger array of nutrients. It will also balance out the toxins you ingest. Everything you eat has toxins of one sort or another, even 'natural' foods.
* Eat slowly and chew thoroughly. Your mum told you this – she was right.
* As we've discussed, do not eat many small meals during the course of the day. Give your body a chance to burn off excess fat by limiting yourself to two or three meals a day.
* Rule of thumb: your diet should be one third raw vegetables and fruit, one third cooked vegetables, one third meat or fish. But remember, this is only a rough guide, not a decree.
* Do not deprive yourself of food. Even if dieting, you will make better progress if you are well nourished.
* Finally, use supplements to ensure sufficient nutrients. But get as much of your nutrition as possible from food.

FOODS TO EAT

Vegetables: Choose colourful, low-starch vegetables such as spinach, cauliflower, celery, broccoli, asparagus, aubergines, greens (iceberg lettuce is not very green), etc.

Meat, fish and eggs: This would include virtually all flesh. My research suggests you need to eat 1.5g of protein per kilogram of body weight daily. That comes to about 75 to 100g of meat or fish in each meal, or up to 425g per day. If that feels like too much, you can reduce your meat and fish bills by taking branched chain amino acids, a dietary supplement that provides about 15g of protein per tablespoon. Here's why protein is so important: Your brain senses how much of it your body requires and prompts you to keep eating until you fulfil that need. This is why a diet lacking protein leads to obesity – your brain will always be telling you to eat more food.

Organic, grass-fed beef, lamb and pork are preferable, as are free-range chicken, turkey and other poultry. Red meat is fine, in moderation, but birds are healthier. Game, if you can find it, is very good and low in fat (healthy meat tends to be expensive). Wild fish, especially salmon, is also good, but all fish are OK. Shellfish is fine, too – I eat a lot of crabs and clams, as did our prehistoric ancestors (if you're allergic, of course, you must avoid them). You should try to eat roughly equal amounts of meat and fish.

Nuts: These include almonds, walnuts and pecans, among others. They do *not* include cashews, which are toxic to eat raw; 'raw' cashews are actually processed, though not roasted, and are high in carbohydrates. Neither should you eat peanuts, which are actually legumes, not nuts. Stay away from seeds, too, which are loaded with toxins and anti-nutrients.

Fruit: Fresh fruits only, no juices. Take care in your portions, as some modern fruits are bred to contain extra sugar. Melons are great; watermelon is excellent since it contains the antioxidant glutathione and its precursors. It may also elevate testosterone, to the benefit of males and females.

Good oils: This is somewhat of a misnomer, because the truth is that no fat is particularly beneficial. I know that olive oil has been described as a healthy food, and in fact it is the only oil I eat. I use it on salads and, in very small quantities, in cooking, mainly for the flavour it imparts. But it doesn't really do much to improve your health, except that it is less bad than all the other oils people use. Remember, we consumed no oils at all even as recently as 100 years ago. If you do cook with olive oil, never allow it to get so hot that it smokes – if it reaches that temperature, it is being oxidised, and free radicals are being formed.

Beyond that, I take an omega-3 fish-oil supplement on days when I don't eat fish. Sometimes I will even take a cod-liver oil capsule. But all the other common kitchen oils – rape, vegetable, corn, palm – are unnecessary. By now most people know to avoid any hydrogenated oils, or products that contain them (such as margarine), because they contain trans fats, which are completely alien to our bodies and harmful.

FOODS TO AVOID

Many of the questions I get on my blog begin, 'Why can't I eat … ?' Here are the most common ones:

Grains: Oh, yes – that dietary staple that the Food Standards Agency esteems so highly. Simply stated, our bodies are not genetically adapted to processing grains. They can result in allergic reactions, high insulin levels (type-2 diabetes has doubled in the last thirty years, as Brits have followed the high-carb, low-fat mantra of the FSA), obesity and digestive disorders. By the way, sweetcorn is a grain, not a vegetable.

Another strong reason for giving up grains is that they contain lectins, a group of plant proteins. After insulin, the most powerful hormone that regulates appetite, energy metabolism and reproduction is leptin. The leptin gene is highly conserved across different species; it is thought to have evolved in primates some four to seven million years ago. As with insulin, you can develop leptin resistance, which is itself a cause of obesity. Lectins are to blame for this (don't be confused by the similar names) and they are particularly abundant in plant and grain seeds.

Given the exalted PR that bread gets in the Bible, it's hard to demonise it. Just remember that your genes were born many millennia before the biblical era and therefore remain unimpressed. Bread is the ultimate poverty food – it exists only because grain is cheap, easy to grow and is less perishable than other foods. Now, in the age of domesticated protein on the hoof and refrigeration, bread has outlived its usefulness. It is an inferior food that has no place in a healthy diet. The same is true of anything made with flour (pasta, baked goods) or other grains (rice, barley, corn). It's fine for herbivorous animals, but not for us humans.

Eating whole grains is slightly healthier than the refined variety, but it's not as good as simply giving them up altogether.

Dairy: We are the only animal that drinks milk into adulthood and consumes another creature's milk. Humans are genetically adapted to mother's milk until weaning, and that is as far as it should go. Also, commercial cow's milk contains excess growth factors such as bovine growth hormone and IGF-1 (insulin-like growth factor) as calves, unlike you, have to grow a lot in a hurry. The processing of milk products creates harmful trans fats.

Some dairy in small amounts is acceptable (like unsweetened yogurt or cheese for flavouring).

Starchy foods: This includes potatoes, which are not vegetables, technically speaking, but tubers – plant forms that specialise in storing energy. It also includes most root vegetables, such as yams, sweet potatoes, parsnips, water chestnuts, turnips and radishes (although some raw carrots or beetroots in moderation are OK). It definitely includes crisps.

Oils and fats: This includes most oils (except for olive), butter and lard, of course. You'll get plenty of fats from the animal protein you eat.

Certain fruits: Bananas or any dried fruit, as they contain too much sugar.

Salt: I will concede that salt is essential and not a toxin. But the level at which we currently consume it is extravagant; daily intake is over 8 grams, whereas it was less than 0.7 grams during the Palaeolithic period. While normal kidneys might be able to handle this overload, many people now develop hypertension because of a defect in their ability to clear that much sodium.

Non-foods: By now this should be a no-brainer. Just because you can eat it doesn't mean it's food. I'm including all those goodies like doughnuts, biscuits, pies, cakes, sweets, ice cream, etc. I know what you're thinking: 'What about on my birthday?' Well, how about living to have a few more! (I suppose a little birthday cake once a year would be sort of OK.)

Certain plant-based foods: Somehow, we have all absorbed the idea that anything that grows in the earth must be healthy to eat. While it's true that most fruits and vegetables are good for us and should be a major part of our diet, there are also plants that promote obesity and make us sick. It's not as though plants *want* us to eat them. They don't really care whether or not you're in good health.

Soy (including soy sauce, tofu and other products made from soy, and that staple of Japanese restaurants, edamame) should be avoided because they are high in lectins and oestrogen. In its natural state, the soybean is not edible. It must be extensively processed to remove toxins. Soybean is also a cause of eczema and dermatitis.

You should also take care not to overindulge in peanuts, which are legumes, not nuts. They contain one of the most carcinogenic toxins known – aflatoxin. Peanut allergies are occasionally fatal, but some soybean allergies can kill, too. Peanut, soybean and legume intolerance tend to be associated. I eat chickpeas, lentils and green beans only in moderation. Some people have trouble digesting them, and lentils have a high carbohydrate content.

All pod-like foods, which includes beans and legumes, are actually seeds of one form or another. If seeds were too tasty and nutritious, the plant world would never have survived this long. There is an evolutionary arms race fought between plants and the animals that eat them. A highly nutritious plant that did not defend itself or its seeds would become extinct. Thus seeds contain many toxins, anti-nutrients such as lectins, chemicals such as plant oestrogens (which chemically castrate the males that eat them), acids that interfere with mineral metabolism or proteins that damage the eater's intestines.

Finally, by dropping grains, beans, legumes and milk, you will shift the pH balance of your food and therefore your body from acidic towards a more neutral and even slightly alkaline state. This is a very good thing. It will permit better mineral metabolism, adding density to your skeletal mass, which is especially important for children's diets. Grains were a major factor in the rickets epidemic in Great Britain, which caused developmental problems with the poor children of the Industrial Revolution – stunted growth, bowed legs, sunken nasal and upper-jaw area of the face, bad teeth and club feet were all symptoms of too little calcium, zinc and protein in the diet of children fed a grain diet.

In our modern times, excess grain intake, too much coffee and phosphoric acid from soft drinks seem to be factors in the eventual loss of bone mass. All these induce an acidic condition that the body buffers by using bone calcium as an antacid.

You can tell the NED is guided by a relatively low-carb philosophy, although not as much as, say, the Atkins diet. People make a giant mistake by calling low-carb diets fads. Eating this way has proven to be healthy, and was an important part of our evolution as a species. To call a diet on which humans lived for millennia a fad is just ignorance. In fact, it is the modern, careless, high-carb, high-grain diet that is the harmful fad.

interlude
How not to eat

WHY MISSING THE OCCASIONAL MEAL IS GOOD FOR YOU

Just as we must learn to eat properly, we should also learn how to *not* eat. For a variety of reasons, none having to do with counting calories, I recommend that you undertake the occasional mini-fast. Once a week or so, you should go a day eating very little or nothing.

That doesn't mean you starve yourself. If you go hungry today, you make up for it tomorrow by eating more. I realise that the idea of skipping a meal or going for a day without food is unsettling to most beginners. One of my blog readers told me this was the most frightening concept to grasp. Having lost some 70 pounds and seeing muscle where there used to be slabs of fat, he has since become a dedicated advocate of intermittent fasting.

Every living creature throughout history has gone hungry now and then. Intermittent fasting is embedded in our metabolism; food scarcity was a normal part of life for our ancestors. The research suggests that prehistoric hunter-gatherers spent about one third of their lives hungry, which is more deprivation than we need for our purposes. But a little self-imposed food scarcity is a good thing.

In fact, our bodies respond to it in an interesting way: brief fasting reduces oxidative stress and improves insulin sensitivity and protein turnover in muscle. A little hunger turns on your body's repair mechanisms. So, doing without the occasional feeding is a powerful way to slow ageing. I skip one dinner a week, chosen at random. On those nights, I go to bed early. You burn fat while you sleep, so the more sleep you get, the leaner you will be. Sometimes I skip breakfast and lunch but enjoy a big dinner.

You may already be aware of the scientific research into calorie restriction (CR) as a way of extending life. The practice has become a small but impassioned global movement. It says, in essence, that if we can manage on 900 to 1,000 calories a day instead of our typical 2,000 to 2,500, we can live significantly longer and in better health. There have been studies in animals and other organisms that suggest calorie restriction can increase longevity. It has been shown to improve health markers in rats, primates and humans.

Because reduced calorie intake lowers the metabolic rate, CR works by protecting against the oxidation of tissues through ROS (reactive oxygen species). It stabilises the cell membranes by reducing their rate of oxidation and by decreasing the polyunsaturated fat content of the membrane. The higher the polyunsaturated fat content of the membrane, the shorter the life span in rats, pigeons and humans. (This surprising news should be a little unsettling to the omega-3 crowd, myself included. I try to balance the polyunsaturated fat content of my cell membranes through periodic fasting and the use of antioxidants. But you can't control everything.)

Here is where I part with the people who do chronic dietary restriction. Aside from the chronic misery of living on so little food, there are other reasons to avoid the CR lifestyle. It seems the stress response itself begins to be the problem, rather than the solution. CR diets affect the brain, which may lose cortical mass with prolonged food deprivation. Anorexics have shrivelled brains, which may be an underlying reason for their inability to recover from their dangerous behaviour. Intermittent fasting protects the brain. Chronic CR, unless practised with high sophistication, may not.

While most of the research has looked at chronic deprivation as an anti-ageing intervention, it is becoming clear that intermittent caloric deprivation may be equally effective. Mild intermittent stressors like fasting and exercise can be enough to increase resistance to disease and improve or extend the quality of life. Eating half your normal intake one day and then one and a half times your normal diet the next is as beneficial as restricting calories every day.

Intermittent fasting can increase the average and maximum life span by 30 to 50 per cent in rodents. It has been found to decrease the incidence of tumours and kidney disease, and can increase resistance to dysfunction and degeneration in stroke and those who suffer with Alzheimer's, Parkinson's and Huntington's diseases. Intermittent fasting enhances resistance to oxidative, metabolic and other types of stress. It is nice to know that our obsession with eating so regularly is so completely wrong. Go ahead and skip that meal, and reap the rewards of better metabolism and enhanced resistance to stress and disease.

The benefits of calorie restriction, we are learning, seem to come primarily from the restriction of glucose in the diet. So, just by eating the diet I recommend, you can achieve the same benefits as CR bestows. And you won't have to go hungry and cranky for the rest of your life.

Experiments with bacteria show that life extension for these one-celled organisms can be gained by switching their fuel from glucose to fat, or by shutting down chronic sugar-burning through anaerobic exercise, which burns out the glycogen in the cell. (Yes, scientists can even make bacteria exercise!) Unfortunately, so far all the research is being done on microbes. I hope they get around to studying it in humans soon.

Here's how cutting out glucose works on your cells. The genes that control ageing and life span do so by signalling over what is known as the insulin-IGF-1 pathway. We're all familiar by now with insulin, the hormone made in the pancreas whose job it is to make nutrients in the blood available to the body. Less well known is IGF-1, a potent anabolic hormone manufactured primarily in the liver that increases cellular metabolism, enhances the function of tissues and helps maintain blood glucose within a healthy range. Together, insulin and IGF-1 control growth and glucose metabolism in humans and other organisms. The economic feedback loop between glucose and life span probably exists in all organisms; insulin/IGF-1 signalling exists in everything from worms to humans.

That connection was critical to us 40,000 years ago, when carbohydrate was a rare nutrient. Glucose – the by-product of carbohydrates – became a valuable internal signal conveying information about our environment. A low glucose flow through the brain's detection circuits would be a clear signal of scarcity; a high flow would be a signal of abundance and a signal that the body should store some of that surplus energy in the form of fat.

The hypothalamus is a brain region that regulates food intake and energy metabolism. Rats with decreased levels of insulin receptors in the hypothalamus eat voraciously and are insulin resistant in other tissues as well. This suggests that insulin signalling in the brain can regulate whole body weight and energy metabolism in a way that is consistent with the ageing effect of insulin-IGF-1 signalling.

Diabetes of the brain, as insulin resistance of the brain is sometimes called, contributes to unhealthy ageing. It promotes overeating, poor glucose control and oxidation in the brain. I have often wondered why some type-2 diabetics I know are so apt to overeat; their hunger is often voracious, even though they store thousands of calories of energy in their fat. They eat as though they have brain damage and, apparently, some or all of them do. The inflammation produced by their elevated blood glucose damages the energy-sensing circuits of the brain. Brain imaging shows that the obese tend to have shrunken brains.

Diabetes of the body may promote diabetes of the brain. The areas of the brain most vulnerable are those associated with the development of Alzheimer's disease. Glucose restriction may protect the body and the brain by turning down the insulin-IGF-1 signalling pathway.

The signal of glucose abundance is also tied to DNA expression. During times of plentiful nutrition, the most effective way for DNA to propagate itself is through reproduction, since there is enough energy out there to support offspring. When there is no excess glucose, DNA is best served by not reproducing. Low levels of insulin and carbohydrate are what send that signal, in which case it is in the DNA's interest to preserve itself for as long as possible through gene repair, stress resistance and cell maintenance. For DNA to self-propagate most efficiently, it has evolved this simple and economic feedback loop.

The existence of this feedback seems to be well established and suggests a number of ways of improving health in humans. That message of glucose scarcity is what we want to send to our bodies, even if a little trickery is required. We want them to focus on gene repair. I choose to live like a wild human rather than a lab rat. I opt for inter-mittent, ad hoc CR, retaining my lean body mass while enjoying, as far as I can see, the full benefits of calorie restriction. I also exercise and, thus, expose my body to another form of CR – an acute negative energy balance. In most things, the wild human is my role model. We would all do better if we relearned how to be good animals.

three
getting started:
the first month

Some of those who already follow the NED tell me they have a bit of trouble in the beginning. They have a difficult time abandoning the idea that they must cut calories and exercise more if they want to lose weight.

When I tell them they ought to focus on making muscle instead of dropping pounds, they begin to understand.

The NED is intended to alter your metabolism to favour muscle and brain tissue over fat. Once people see that proper eating and exercise can achieve that goal, the programme begins to make sense. They learn to focus on body composition – the balance of muscle versus fat – instead of calories or weight, and give up the idea that they have to starve in order to lose pounds.

I have a lot of muscle, which raises my resting energy expenditure. I burn 300 to 365 more calories every day than the average person my age even when I'm doing nothing (something I do quite a lot). This difference translates to about ten pounds of fat per year. I also expend more energy when I do play or exercise, and I am active throughout the day because I can do things most people my age cannot.

I eat an unbelievable amount of food and never gain weight. Here, for example, is today's intake. Breakfast: half a ham steak cooked in a pan, three cooked egg whites, half a cantaloupe. Lunch: a huge salad of romaine (cos) lettuce, raw broccoli, cauliflower, red cabbage, kalamata olives, half an avocado and about nine ounces of smoked salmon, dressed with balsamic vinegar and olive oil. Dinner: half a rack of barbecued pork ribs, asparagus sautéed in garlic and olive oil, and half a red pepper grilled with the ribs. Not exactly starvation.

The people who do have a problem when starting the NED are likely to be those who had the unhealthiest diets before. Some people continue to experience serious sugar cravings. To them, I recommend a gram of branched chain amino acid. It will decrease your craving for sweets because the liver will convert this amino acid to glucose in the amount your body needs (but no more).

Other people start the diet with low magnesium stores, which can lead to cramping, fatigue, brain fade, heart palpitations and oedema (swelling and water retention), all harmless possible side effects of the plan. To prevent that, I suggest two to four weeks of magnesium supplements before starting and during the first month – 500mg of magnesium oxide or citrate, twice a day. As always, check with your doctor first. If you have a history of renal insufficiency or other disorders, taking magnesium pills could result in levels that are too high. But for most healthy people, magnesium may help in the diet's early days.

The main problem with any diet that restricts what you eat is compliance. Most dieters cheat or stop. They do so because they are hungry and their brains are lacking glucose. A brain suffering a crisis in its supply of glucose has no willpower*. In other words, a traditional diet makes it harder for you to resist carbs and sugar, not easier.

The other problem is monotony. Diets require too much regimentation, too much work and thought. They bore you.

These are not problems on the NED because it does not restrict calories, and the food is delicious and satisfying. There is no routine or boredom because variation and randomness are part of the strategy. I surveyed my website readers and found some who have been following the diet for fifteen years. I have been on it for at least twenty-five years. It is a way of life.

By the end of the first week, you will probably have lost about five pounds. You will appear less puffy and the pinkness in your face will lessen, signs that you are less inflamed. You

---

* See Matthew T. Gailliot and Roy F. Baumeister, 'The Physiology of Willpower: Linking Blood Glucose to Self-Control' Personality and Social Psychology Review, 2007; 11; 303 and Zheng and Berthoud. Neural Systems Controlling the Drive to Eat: Mind Versus Metabolism. Physiology (2008) vol. 23 (2) pp. 75–83.

should be sleeping better, burning plenty of fat as you sleep, and feel less fatigued.

Some brightening of mood usually occurs because the energy and nutrients meant for your brain are no longer being siphoned off by your fat. People usually tell me they feel less stressed, more peaceful. The reason is that their hormones are adjusting; they no longer release a big burst of insulin after eating, which sends blood glucose crashing an hour later in a person who has impaired metabolism (the pancrease does not release glucagon to offset the fall in serum glucose). The brain responds to a glucose crash by releasing stress hormones that raise blood pressure and elevate feelings of anxiety.

I have come to the conclusion that many people develop a conditioned fear of starvation through repeated glucose crashes. The stress hormones increase the intensity of the crash, and each incident imbeds the memory more deeply in the metabolic networks. Stress hormones in the presence of insulin make you eat more, and your preferences are for fat and sugar. Your cravings are not a sign of psychological weakness – they have physiological origins.

As you will see, it really is easy to begin this eating plan. There are just a few things to master, which will be easily learned in one week.

First, make a list of the appalling things you have been eating. I won't list them: you know what they are. Note especially how many grams of carbohydrates you take in. Keep the list as a reminder of how far off track one can get through habit and lack of consideration. Now you're ready to eat and exercise.

Week One

MONDAY

Breakfast: Have some salmon – smoked, canned or fresh with spices. Eat some fresh celery and some melon. Celery is a great source of fibre and will raise your testosterone, which is beneficial to males and females. Melon is a good source of minerals and antioxidants.

Lunch: Have a big fresh salad topped with prawns, roast turkey or grilled chicken and full of vegetables such as broccoli, cabbage, green onions, artichoke hearts or palm hearts. Add half an avocado and use olive oil with wine or balsamic vinegar as a dressing.

Dinner: Have some barbecued beef or pork ribs with no sauce. Add a big helping of asparagus and a romaine cos salad to start. Eat no later than 7 p.m. If you can't eat before then, have a snack instead of a meal, perhaps a few slices of lean turkey breast with half an avocado. Have some nuts if you still don't feel satisfied.

Exercise: Learn the abdominal brace. Stand tall and bend slightly forward from the hips as you feel the erector muscles tighten in your lower back. Hold them flexed and stand straight. Then, holding that position, push your stomach out a bit. Then, lift your heart and look out over your cheek-bones as you walk, not at the ground. This is a position of power that protects and strengthens the spine and lets you see the world in a different way.

TUESDAY

Breakfast: Have an omelette (two eggs, one yolk) with well-cooked and drained bacon, fresh fruit and black coffee. Drink water as needed.

Lunch: Italian … but how can you eat Italian without carbs? I did it for two weeks in Italy just by passing on the bread and pasta, the *primi piatti*. Find a restaurant that serves real Italian-style vegetables. Send the bread back, have a salad and fish or seafood with vegetables. Try to get grilled red peppers with courgettes drenched in olive oil. Drink fresh water with lemon and have a cup of espresso, plain with no sugar or cream.

Dinner: Have a flank steak or rump steak done on the grill. This cut is very lean and contains ample protein. I marinate mine in a teriyaki sauce that I buy at the supermarket. We are not trying to literally live in the Ice Age, just to emulate aspects of that diet, taking our tastes and what is available in stores into account. Just sear a lean flank steak on both sides and cook it until it is red to pink (to your taste) in the centre. Cut up some squash and red peppers, drop them in the marinade for a moment or drizzle a bit of olive oil over them and cook on the grill with the steak. A glass of wine to go with it is fine.

Exercise: Establish your balance in bare feet. Stand tall; settle the weight into your hips and into your feet just before the heels. Lift one foot and shift your weight to the other. Notice how much you sway. Maintain balance on the ball and heel of the foot and by flexing your hip muscles. Good balance can be learned and makes you move gracefully and in safety. Your posture and movement can take years off your appearance. Learn to stand and walk like you are proud of your body.

WEDNESDAY

Breakfast: Half a ham steak with two hard-boiled egg whites and cantaloupe with coffee and plenty of water. Let your hunger determine the size of your portions. Eat all you want but no more.

Lunch: Have two fish tacos with cabbage and fresh salsa, and drink water or unsweetened iced tea. Don't worry about the tortilla – eat as much of it as you need to get the fish and cabbage into your mouth and leave the rest. Or, forget the tortilla and eat with a fork. No rice or beans. A beer is OK, but it will raise your insulin and tell your liver to convert the carbs into fat. Just know the price of what you consume and make your own choices. I find that beer leaves a heavy feeling after a meal, and I hate that.

Dinner: How hungry are you right now, truly? At night I often eat only a salad with smoked salmon, red cabbage, garlic, celery, kalamata olives and avocado. I add a smoked anchovy or two. The bulk will fill you and the nutrition is excellent. You can use any canned seafood you like (canned crab is excellent, although fresh is even better).

Exercise: Start your day with a walk in the briskness of the morning and enjoy the chill. Don't wear a jacket, just dress lightly in shirt and shorts if possible. Your metabolism will thank you and your under-utilised brown adipose (fat) tissues will fire up – these are good at burning calories from other fat. If you feel up to it, sprint lightly a couple of times during your walk.

THURSDAY

Breakfast: Try four hard-boiled eggs, but cut out two of the yolks. Eat some fresh fruit of your choice.

Lunch: If you have time, take a walk for lunch and along the way find a sandwich shop that has good pastrami and coleslaw. Leave just enough bread crust to hold the contents of the sandwich. Or, throw all the bread away and eat the fillings with your fingers. Have unsweetened iced tea or water to drink. After you eat, continue strolling; it is a walk interrupted by food, not really a break. But neither is it a 'power' walk or a rushed one. The walk is to relax, look around at the people and scenery, and to plan your afternoon.

Dinner: You will be hungry by now if you are like me. It is time for a large swordfish steak with a great salad. A glass of pinot grigio goes well with this meal. Before the meal and for the whole afternoon after that salty lunch, drink plenty of water. You might have a bit of cheesecake if you can find a dry one with little or no crust.

Exercise: At work, climb a flight of stairs; drive from the hip and raise your foot high as you climb. Begin standing whenever you take phone calls. Your call will be shorter and more to the point. Do some sprinting when you get home from work before supper. Or play football with your children. A bit of exercise before eating increases insulin sensitivity.

FRIDAY

Friday can be a busy, stressful day. You handle stress better if you eat less, so have a light breakfast of nuts and fruit.

Almonds, walnuts or mixed nuts are preferred. If salted, it should be sea salt and lightly at that.

Lunch: I suggest a salad of vegetables, lettuce and plenty of celery, with some chicken or seafood.

Dinner: Wide open. Just make good choices, send the bread back, kill the croutons, and choose your meal wisely from vegetables, seafood and lean meat. Try not to eat carbohydrates with fat. That means you will have to skip the potatoes and gravy and have vegetables instead.

Exercise: Just do the posture routine and play at your balance in the morning or at work for a break. For activity, practise walking in the office, campus or warehouse – wherever you work – with your new posture while doing the abdominal brace. Lift your heart and look over your cheekbones as you walk. I bet you get some compliments.

SATURDAY

If you plan to skip dinner tonight, have a large breakfast and judge the size of your lunch by your hunger. By now, you should have some leftovers from your previous meals; I always have plenty in the refrigerator because we cook lots of food and then put the rest away. It makes a very convenient, fast breakfast. Also, keep a dozen hard-boiled eggs and some lean turkey breast in the fridge for a quick meal or snack. Don't go chronically hungry; eat these leftovers and nuts and celery.

Breakfast: Rather than having the carb-laden meals people usually enjoy for breakfast, you're eating your leftovers from dinner the night before, along with fresh fruit with coffee. Meats and seafood from previous meals make the best, quickest breakfasts.

Lunch: Canned or packaged smoked salmon or tuna in a salad with vegetables such as red cabbage, broccoli, tomato, cauliflower, celery, kalamata olives, fresh garlic and spring onions. Olive oil and balsamic vinegar for dressing, with fresh basil sprinkled on top. Use whatever appeals to you.

Dinner: Skip it and don't eat until Sunday morning. Most of you will probably anticipate this with some fear and so you'll load up at lunch. This is OK, but you will get over it and eventually will randomise your meal-skipping so even you can't anticipate the next time you'll go hungry. The long interval between meals turns on genes that delay the ageing process and turns off the insulin-IGF-1 pathway that ages you. If you have some trouble with dizziness or feel ravenously hungry, those are signs that your metabolism has been damaged by years of carbohydrate abuse. Just take a gram of branched amino acid supplements and remind yourself that your ancestors endured many episodes of hunger, and that your metabolism is designed to deal with brief fasts.

Exercise: During your fasting period, take a walk at dinner-time. If you are used to taking exercise as an experienced weightlifter, go to the gym and do a solid workout. When you fast, you have to use your muscles to retain their protein. Activity is a signal to your metabolism to retain muscle even in the face of an energy shortage. You will release growth hormone to mobilise fat to fuel your exercise and the by-product of fat metabolism will supply ketones to the brain. A workout with weights will release lactate as fuel for the brain. Your brain will have adequate substitutes for glucose from these sources, so you may even find that you are not hungry at all.

SUNDAY

If you skipped dinner on Saturday, make sure you eat well on Sunday. You won't be ravenous since you are now using fat as energy; your brain is nourished and feeding on ketones from the fat you burn.

Breakfast: Fresh fruit and a scrambled egg.

Lunch: A large lunch is in order. I suggest fish such as fresh salmon or tuna (grill some extra for tomorrow's breakfast or a quick snack) over broccoli and celery drizzled with olive oil and balsamic vinegar, sprinkled with fresh garlic and Asian red chillies. The omega-3 oils in the fish will reduce the inflammation from toxins that may be released as the fat cells you are losing release their contents.

Dinner: I would have steak Romano covered with grilled prawns in a garlic and lemon sauce along with sautéed asparagus and banana squash done on the grill. Cut the squash into strips and grill them until they soften and become slightly translucent. Grill the steak and then put sauce and steamed asparagus over the top. Lay the prawns around the steak and pour sauce on them, too. To make the sauce, melt some Romano cheese with a bit of flavoured olive oil. Grilled squash is a great substitute for chips (the colour is similar), but you will lose your taste for potatoes soon and never want to go back.

Exercise: Before dinner, think about what you did to raise your insulin sensitivity during the day. Do something to raise it before you eat. One nice way is to hug your partner and, if you can, lift them carefully off the ground, or move something you have been meaning to relocate or get rid of. Pick up a small child and walk around the house. Climb the stairs, or play with your children or dogs. I love to shoot baskets in the driveway for a few minutes, but I love picking up my wife more.

AFTER YOUR FIRST WEEK

On Monday morning you will be getting compliments or stares from slightly envious friends in the office. You will look and feel younger and stronger. You will have more energy because your brain is well fed and your mitochondria, those little energy furnaces in all your cells, will begin to regenerate as you relieve the glucose assault to which they have been subjected.

At this point, the sabotage may begin. Your friends will have noticed that you are eating in what they consider to be a strange way. It always happens. Don't bother to explain your appearance or eating to them since they will only argue with you to bring you back to eating the way *they* feel comfortable with.

Every female I know who has followed the diet has experienced this. When we were dating, my wife lost five dress sizes in a matter of a few months and her co-workers started saying, 'You're too skinny,' and brought her candy and doughnuts in the morning. They were trying to undermine her, I think. It will happen to guys in the gym as well; you will hear that you have to drink energy drinks and protein shakes and 'do your cardio' – aerobic exercise. It is all nonsense.

I do not specify portion size anywhere in this eating plan. Nobody but you knows what your appetite and energy expenditures are. So why would they attempt to tell you how much you should eat? Once your metabolism is healed, your appetite will become a healthy guide to your energy intake. I have weighed 14 stone for over 50 years and I have never counted my calorific intake or my energy expenditures. Nor do I use anything other than my appetite to limit how much I eat.

The low-energy density of the NED and the filling nature of the food (it is nearly impossible to overeat), mixed with the occasional brief fast, are more than enough to manage your energy intake. As your body composition improves, your appetite will determine your eating appropriately.

Week Two

MONDAY

Breakfast: Slices of avocado, lean turkey breast, slices of apple and grapes.

Lunch: Prawns or canned fresh tuna mixed with olives, leeks and big chunks of celery drizzled with olive oil and flavoured vinegar.

Dinner: Lean flank steak, marinated lightly in barbecue sauce and grilled with red pepper. If you feel as though you've been eating too much red meat, feel free to replace it with skinless chicken breast or even pork chops. As a vegetable, steam or sauté broccoli or asparagus. Be creative and cook extra for breakfast or lunch another day.

Exercise: Lift weights at the gym or at home. Or, sprint in a field or on a stationary bike. If you use a bike with a speedometer or energy meter, see how many watts you can generate in a gentle but maximum effort, or how far and fast you pedal. Then try to exceed that two more times.

TUESDAY

Breakfast: Eggs scrambled with bits of Italian sausage, tomato and mushrooms. Add a large slice of honeydew melon with a few dark red grapes.

Lunch: Mozzarella cheese chunks, lean turkey breast over lettuce topped with tomatoes, black olives and celery with Caesar dressing. Don't use a dressing with hydrogenated oil.

Dinner: Salmon steak grilled or blackened with red peppers and celery, topped with slices of avocado and hot chillies. Make a large coleslaw salad with raw red and white cabbage mixed with wine vinegar and olive oil and a few chilli flakes.

Exercise: Lie on your back in a field or your garden and look up at the sky. Just do nothing as you watch the clouds or stars. (Reading or watching television is not doing nothing.)

WEDNESDAY

Breakfast: Leftover flank steak or salmon from Monday or Tuesday. Have a small bunch of red grapes.

Lunch: Sauerkraut with two large, grilled frankfurters. I know that hotdogs are supposed to be toxic, but I love them. The large ones taste much better than the small ones, which I keep around as a quick snack.

Dinner: When our local shop has lobster or fresh crab, we buy them. Serve with a tomato and mozzarella salad with thin red onion slices and basil and olive oil. Top it off with coffee and cheesecake.

Exercise: If you have children, buy a thick, soft rope eight to twelve feet long. Take them to a field and play tug-of-war. When I do this with my grandchildren, every kid in the park comes over to help my grandchildren try and beat me. I end up with a good workout, and the kids love it.

THURSDAY

Breakfast: Omelette cooked with onion or leftover broccoli or asparagus. A few slices of bacon, well cooked and drained. Add a handful of red raspberries or any fresh fruit of the season.

Lunch: A few fresh prawns with celery slices and a bit of tomato and red onion salad and avocado drizzled lightly with olive oil and flavoured vinegar.

Dinner: Grill a pork and beef skewer with red onion and red peppers. Steam two stems of broccoli and have a large salad with romaine cos lettuce, avocado, celery and olives in creamy Italian dressing.

Exercise: Take a medicine ball outside and toss it as high up as you can. Move out of the way as it falls. Then, throw it as far forward as you can and sprint after it. Then throw it sideways, sprint to it and throw it back over your head (careful with this – don't use your lower back as a hinge, but stay straight, bend at the hips and use your legs).

FRIDAY

Breakfast: Two thin pork chops grilled in a pan with fresh rosemary. A few slices of watermelon are refreshing with this, or try cantaloupe.

Lunch: Fresh or canned tuna chunks over lettuce and tomatoes, sprinkled with sliced spring onions and a creamy Italian dressing. Or, use your fresh coleslaw as a bed under the fish.

Dinner: Salmon steak grilled in a pan with celery, olives, broccoli and slices of leek, mushrooms and red chillies. Use a lemon sauce.

Exercise: Practise the abdominal brace and take a walk, preferably in the cool air so you get just a hint of chill. Cold has some benefits of exercise.

SATURDAY

Breakfast: Leftover pork chop from Friday with cantaloupe slices and a few red grapes.

Lunch: Have a handful of unsalted mixed nuts with a bit of Jarlsberg cheese. If you get hungry before dinner, take 500mg of leucine.

Dinner: Have a huge plate of steamed mussels with artichoke hearts sautéed in olive oil with a big salad of mixed greens, bok choy slices, olives and chunks of avocado.

Exercise: Go for a brief walk or climb a few flights of stairs.

SUNDAY

Breakfast: Bacon and egg-white omelette with fruit.

Lunch: Small prawn cocktail with avocado and celery drizzled with olive oil and flavoured vinegar.

Dinner: A large steak with sautéed spinach. A romaine cos salad with thin slices of white onion and almond slices, topped with an anchovy in Italian dressing.

Exercise: Before dinner, hike in the wildest park you can find.

Week Three

MONDAY

Breakfast: Ground beef with scrambled eggs and cheese with some grapes and blueberries.

Lunch: Home-made egg salad with red onion slices, black and green olives over romaine with your favourite salad dressing. Have a few cantaloupe slices.

Dinner: Barbecued spare ribs with a steamed fresh artichoke.

Exercise: Lift weights at the gym or at home.

TUESDAY

Breakfast: Two hard-boiled eggs, slices of avocado, Jarlsberg cheese, and cantaloupe with a few red grapes.

Lunch: A light salad with celery, red cabbage, red onion and avocado and canned crab or tuna.

Dinner: Let's eat out. Steak Oscar – a grilled steak covered with crab in a Béarnaise sauce and asparagus with a Caesar salad.

Exercise: Sprint for 10 seconds on a stationary bike, then pedal smoothly for 20 to 30 seconds, and then sprint a bit harder for another 10 seconds. Do this about half a dozen times, sprinting a bit harder each time, until you are maxing out by the last sprint (I assume you have your doctor's clearance to exercise). Heart patients are rehabilitated with high-intensity (but brief) training. It is far safer, and more effective, than jogging.

WEDNESDAY

Breakfast: A few of the leftover barbecued ribs with fresh cantaloupe slices and a few red grapes for colour.

Lunch: Fresh or packaged smoked salmon over fresh spinach, green olives, romaine cos lettuce, celery and tomato with pine nuts sprinkled over.

Dinner: Fresh steamed mussels in a red marinara sauce with a steamed artichoke and an olive oil and balsamic vinegar dip with hot chilli bits.

Exercise: Lift weights or just do nothing for half an hour, lying on your back, gazing at the ceiling or sky.

THURSDAY

Breakfast: Skip breakfast, or just have some leftovers.

Lunch: Heart of romaine with freshly cooked bacon, anchovies, grated Romano cheese, olives, tomato and red chilli flakes topped with Italian dressing.

Dinner: A large swordfish steak grilled in olive oil and garlic with broccoli, red cabbage, celery, fresh white mushrooms and spring onion. A small mixed green salad with avocado and thin slices of raw carrot.

Exercise: Shoot baskets before dinner or walk up several flights of stairs at work or at home.

FRIDAY

Breakfast: Bacon leftovers from the previous lunch with a slice of cantaloupe with slices of avocado and a few red grapes.

Lunch: Fresh chicken breast on sliced tomatoes and onions with dressing.

Dinner: Eat out and have fresh crab with a salad.

Exercise: Nothing at all.

SATURDAY

Breakfast: Watermelon, red grapes, a frankfurter sliced and scrambled with two eggs.

Lunch: Turkey breast over fresh spinach, sprinkled with tomato slices, red onions, leeks and hot green chillies with a few slices of fresh strawberries for colour.

Dinner: Sirloin steak with a great vegetable like leeks grilled with banana squash.

Exercise: Stand up during the commercials when you watch TV. Begin to adopt that as a habit. Sitting is not just 'not exercising'. Prolonged sitting is damaging because it interrupts fat metabolism.

SUNDAY

Breakfast: Pear and watermelon with sliced, lean turkey breast.

Lunch: Frozen cooked prawn, thawed but cold, with tomatoes, red onions, leeks, a bit of kale and two stalks of celery with dark olives. Dressing to taste.

Dinner: A large pork loin cooked on the barbecue. Add a large mixed green salad with raw red cabbage slices, tomato and big chunks of very fresh celery.

Exercise: Get some exposure to cold or sunshine. Cold exposure is exercise. Sunshine helps to produce vitamin D.

Week Four

MONDAY

Breakfast: Leftover pork loin with cantaloupe. (I may eat as much as ten ounces of lean pork loin at breakfast.)

Lunch: A home-made fish or chicken taco topped with romaine lettuce with slices of fresh red and white cabbage and slices of jalapeno, all on a large tortilla lightly burned in a pan.

Dinner: One of the often-repeated meals: spare ribs on the grill with artichokes and a romaine cos salad.

Exercise: Take up a sport long neglected, or start one you've always wanted to try – preferably one that makes you move, like basketball or tennis.

TUESDAY

Breakfast: Eggs with bacon, a few grapes and half a pear.

Lunch: Chunks of grilled, leftover pork loin over mixed salad greens sprinkled with slices of leeks and topped with slices of celery and olives with olive oil and a little balsamic vinegar. Sprinkle with dried chilli pieces.

Dinner: Lightly grilled cod over a bed of lettuce with prawns and steamed broccoli.

Exercise: If you haven't already, join a gym and start weight training.

WEDNESDAY

Breakfast: Three small, thin pork chops sautéed in olive oil with thin slices of white onion and slices of honeydew melon and apple.

Lunch: One can of smoked oysters over lettuce with snow peas and sliced green olives with jalapeno and flecks of red chilli.

Dinner: Large cooked, packaged prawns with avocado slices over a bed of romaine cos lettuce and kale. (We like to serve it with olive oil and balsamic vinegar for dressing and Marie Rose sauce on the side.)

Exercise: Kick a ball around with a child or friend.

THURSDAY

Breakfast: Two hard-boiled eggs, two slices of well-cooked drained bacon with a few fresh strawberries and grapes.

Lunch: Grilled chicken breast with a salad of romaine cos lettuce, artichoke hearts, red cabbage with bits of bacon and creamy Italian dressing.

Dinner: Egg drop soup made with chicken broth into which you put some spinach, tomato and bits of crab meat. Alongside that, stir-fry broccoli and sliced beef with hot chillies and a light teriyaki sauce.

Exercise: Second session of weight training. Focus on learning the equipment and the basic exercises from an instructor. Forget what they tell you about how to eat. Don't 'do your cardio', as they may suggest.

FRIDAY

Breakfast: Almonds and avocado with three hard-boiled eggs. Eat just one or two of the yolks.

Lunch: Sliced beef in a romaine cos salad sprinkled with cheese slices, tomato and red onion slices. We buy pre-cooked, packaged beef and use it often in salads for lunch or with fruit for breakfast.

Dinner: Halibut sautéed and placed hot over fresh spinach to cook it. Sautéed asparagus seasoned with flakes of red chillies to taste with a large heart of romaine cos salad with palm hearts and olives.

Exercise: Do nothing.

SATURDAY

Breakfast: A ham steak lightly grilled with a few slices of watermelon, a piece of pear and a few red grapes.

Lunch: Smoked turkey breast (keep handy in the refrigerator for a quick meal or occasional snack) with avocado.

Dinner: Buy a pre-cooked whole chicken just off the grill and take it home to serve with any fresh vegetables that look good that day in the store.

Exercise: Take an easy walk in the morning when it's cool to chilly (don't wrap up).

SUNDAY

Breakfast: Leftover chicken with avocado slices.

Lunch: Prawns over lettuce, with hard-boiled egg slices, celery, green olive and artichoke heart salad.

Dinner: Skip dinner (optional).

Exercise: Walk easily for twenty minutes instead of eating.

If you think about the challenges our ancestors faced, it will help you realise that what some fitness experts see as motivational problems are actually evolved adaptations. Recognition and acceptance of this will go a long way towards helping you make healthy changes.

The fact that you are alive is a remarkable thing. The odds against it are great. The genes you carry contain information from a continuous strand of surviving organisms that extends two billion years back in time. You are an improbable event and your existence is testimony to the toughness and adaptability of the ancestral line whence you come. You are a survivor, well equipped to live and thrive. Recognise, however, that the world for which your genes encoded a successful design does not exist today.

Your brain and body expect you to live a life of movement and action, of challenge and response, of variety and adaptation. Your brain still 'sees' sensory inputs as though you are a hunter-gatherer and, at the instinctive level, directs your actions accordingly.

Variety and play are the essential human attributes. By keeping your workouts brief and exhilarating you won't get bored. By adding lots of outdoor activity and play, you will enjoy the power and fitness you gain. If you start a new sport, or pick up one long neglected, you will see how the power you gain improves your play. The feedback between the training and your new power in the sport will be habit-forming.

I fail to see how anyone can train five or six days a week in the gym and for hours at a time. That is factory or agricultural work, not anything human beings were evolved to do. And the paradox is that you will gain less strength and fitness if you over-train. You will join the thousands who quit exercising out of sheer boredom.

As for goals, don't set any. The ones you are likely to choose are not functional. You will say, 'I want to lose x pounds', but you really want to lose fat, not lean body mass. You actually want to *gain* lean body mass.

You can't control the outcome, only the process. Just accept that what you are doing is what your body and mind were designed to do, and that this active and metabolically challenging lifestyle is how it is going to be from now on.

interlude
the worst food known to man

I have strong views on how to eat because it is crucial to health. But I try not to demonise particular foods, even very bad ones. I tend to be a libertarian in these matters; you should know the facts, then make your own choices. I despise diets that dictate to adults what they may and may not eat, partly because ultimately those regimens fail, but also because I dislike rigid authoritarianism in general.

However, I am deeply concerned with how people feed their children. Many of my website members keep their children on the diet and get wonderfully positive results. My wife and I feed our grandchildren the same food we eat and they love it and don't want to go home.

But not everyone treats children this way. There is one dish in particular that is beloved by juvenile palates and is ubiquitous in the modern youthful diet. It is, in my view, the absolute worst food a human being can eat.

A few years ago, my wife and I were having an early supper at one of her favourite restaurants, a place called the Cheesecake Factory. (It is a testament to the ease with which one can follow our diet that you can find plenty to eat at a place with such a name.) We shared the artichoke appetiser, which was steamed and then grilled with a balsamic and olive oil dip, and we split a Caesar salad. We each also had the combination steak Diane and crusted salmon entrée with asparagus on the side and enjoyed a glass of pinot grigio. No bread, no croutons.

I looked over to my right and saw a family of seven sitting down to a big mound of brown food. That was the only colour on the table. A bad sign. Colour is a reliable guide to beautiful, well-balanced meals. The more colours on the table, and the brighter they are, the better the eating.

The family included all ages, from grandfather to small children. The mound was mostly made up of chips, which covered nearly all of every plate. The monochromatic meal was interrupted only by the dark brown of a hamburger here and there, the light brown of bread, and the blackish-brown of the colas they were drinking.

The sight ruined my dinner.

I am used to seeing children being fed chips by their parents. It is a cheap dish. It appears to be a vegetable (although it is actually a tuber). Kids love it, and so it is always on the children's menu, no matter where you go. Nearly every kiddie meal at a fast-food restaurant features chips and a toy, giving potatoes yet another happy association in the mind of a child. Children today have a Pavlovian response to chips – they signify dining out amid familial love and toys and pleasant experiences.

They also mean big trouble. A chip is nothing but a ship of carbs carrying a load of grease. I think a combined carb-fat load must have been an extremely rare event in the nutritional history of our species. In ancestral times of 100,000 years ago, fat would have accompanied protein, as in meat – not a simple carb. I don't think our metabolism really knows how to handle the combination. Our metabolic networks must be stressed by this mixed signal. The carbs release insulin, which shuts down fat-burning. The high fat load and high blood sugar that results become a heavy sludge in the bloodstream, bruising the blood vessel lining, the epithelium. The release of insulin also opens the epithelium to the intrusion of fats. These fats are then oxidised, driven by the inflammatory response to high blood glucose. Oxidising fat on a stream of glucose-mediated free radicals inflames the vasculature (circulatory system), promoting cardiovascular disease. The liver is confused, I think, when it senses high insulin, blood glucose and high fat: how should it respond to this unusual signal?

I really hate it when I see a kid eating chips. I love my grandchildren too much to buy chips for them. I hope they learn to associate vegetables and good food with their Pa-Pa. When I take them out, I let them order from the adult menu. It is costly because I have a lot of grandchildren, but it is worth it to teach them what good food is like.

four
How to exercise

Today is a gym day for me. I'd like you to come along.

I visit here anywhere between once and four times a week. It depends completely on how I feel. If I worked out hard last time, I may need two or three days off to recover. It also varies because I want to keep my workouts a little random and unplanned. Too much regimentation in exercise is a bad thing, regardless of what you've been led to believe.

I spend as little time as possible working out, usually no more than half an hour or so. That's all anybody needs. I also keep my visits to a minimum to avoid boredom. There are nicer places to be and finer things to do with your life than hang around gyms. It's possible to exercise too much.

Here's another good reason to keep your workouts short: the physical stress causes the release of adrenaline, which mobilises fat for burning. But if the exertion goes on too long, the body will release another stress hormone, cortisol, which we don't want, at least not now (it will be released, moderately, later on to help heal the exhausted muscles). This all makes perfect evolutionary sense, since stresses 40,000 years ago tended to be of the short-term 'fight or flight' variety, where adrenaline was essential.

I'm here in the morning, not long after I've wakened, for the simple reason that a workout is more effective if done on an empty stomach. You burn more fat this way. Maybe I'll have a cup of coffee first, since the caffeine starts the adrenaline flowing, increases heart rate, and mobilises fat for burning. But nothing more.

That, too, runs counter to what you may have been taught. The idea that you should first eat – the 'experts' usually counsel a big helping of carbs, supposedly to fuel your muscles – is actually counterproductive if burning off fat is among your goals. Later I'll explain why it is better not only to exercise hungry, but also to put off eating afterwards for up to an hour.

The main goal here is to reach for intensity. I don't want this to sound scary, but each workout needs to take you to an extreme. Your body should be required to do something it has never done before. I've seen people who turn the gym into a routine as predictable as any other, like a task they can do on autopilot. They don't realise they need to push themselves, so they settle for a mildly taxing session that pretty much replicates all the workouts that came before.

That defeats the entire purpose of being here. You should be looking for an experience that will change you, inside and out. Each workout is supposed to leave its mark on you, alter you – to make you a better specimen of human being than you were when you walked in the door. And that's only possible if your exertions reach the point of intensity.

That doesn't mean you need to devote a great deal of time to exercising, however. Professor James Timmons, of Heriot-Watt University in Edinburgh, tested the effect of what he termed 'high-intensity interval training' on the metabolisms of sedentary male volunteers. He said, 'The risk of developing cardiovascular disease and type-2 diabetes is substantially reduced through regular physical activity. Unfortunately, many people feel they simply don't have the time to follow current exercise guidelines. What we have found is that doing a few intense muscle exercises, each lasting only about thirty seconds, dramatically improves your metabolism in just two weeks.' Precisely my point.

First thing I do at the gym is head for a stationary bike. You need to warm up your heart before the real work begins. You don't want to start your day with a heart attack. The second goal here is to warm up everything else, too – to increase my core temperature. When I do that, the pituitary gland responds by releasing growth hormone. That event is vital to a successful workout: the hormone mobilises fat to burn for the rest of my session, and even beyond.

Unlike most people here, however, I won't be on the bike for long – just six minutes total, which is enough time to break a sweat and get a good burn going, if you ride as I do. First, I'll pedal with low resistance at a fast sprint. After one minute of that, I turn the resistance up to the maximum possible, and ride just as hard as I can for the next sixty seconds. I repeat that pattern twice more – a minute of sprinting at low resistance, followed by one that feels as though I am riding through peanut butter. During that sixth minute, I do my best to max out the meter that measures watts of energy expended. Then I'm done.

Professor Timmons's research actually showed that doing just seven minutes *per week* on a stationary bike, riding intensely as I do, can make significant improvements in your ability to metabolise glucose. It's the intensity that counts, not the duration.

Anyway, enough warm-up. Time to move along.

*

The very idea of exercise is alien and unnatural to every life form, us included. No wonder we have such a hard time with it. Either we do too little, or we do it badly – even to the point of harming ourselves with an activity meant to be beneficial.

Perhaps that's because it *is* such an artificial pursuit. I don't mean to say that exertion is unnatural. It is what we are built to do. Our genes are adapted to an existence of hard physical work, and when we fulfil that potential properly they reward us by expressing themselves in a healthy way.

But remember that from an evolutionary perspective humans are lazy overeaters. We survived as a species only by exerting ourselves as little as possible (and thereby conserving energy, back when it was scarce). For most of the time we've existed, our environment has been challenging enough to keep us strenuously active. Thanks to civilisation, the world has changed a great deal since our genes stopped evolving. But even all the labour-saving technology we've invented is a mixed blessing: by solving one set of problems, we created another.

So these are the questions facing us today: how do we motivate an essentially lazy genotype to exert itself? And what form should our exertions take?

As always, we can look back and deduce what kinds of activity our prehistoric forebears practised. Then we can attempt to replicate that activity here and now.

There is no doubt that the hunter-gatherers were strong, stronger than we are. Their remains are very revealing. Cro-Magnon and Neanderthal man left extremely robust skeletons, with huge attachment points for the muscles, which implies exceptional strength. The bones are dense and highly mineralised. The poor Neanderthal has a skeleton that resembles that of a rodeo cowboy, full of injuries and evidence of arthritis from repetitive injury stress, including breaks that healed. Neanderthals must have lived up close with the animals they hunted, because they only had heavy spears that were suitable for thrusting rather than throwing. Cro-Magnons, on the other hand, left behind a taller, less robust skeleton that is relatively free of injuries. It is known that they had spears they could throw, and even implements that would propel the spear farther. And, at some point, they used bows and arrows too.

We can also look to contemporary hunter-gatherer tribes for evidence of ancient activity patterns.

Until the introduction of snowmobiles and rifles, the Eskimo went hunting for seals and whales in traditional ways. First came many hours of quiet exploration and searching, followed by intense moments of the kill. Even butchering and hauling the prey back to camp required brute strength and aerobic capacity.

There are compelling stories of the American Indian's physical exertions. They lived off buffalo and ate on average four pounds of meat a day. They hunted in two ways: they ran the buffalo off cliffs, or rode horses and speared them. The Spanish explorer Vasco da Gama wrote of meeting a Native American Indian who was allegedly seven feet tall and powerfully muscled and could run alongside buffalo to spear them. The American Indian was so beautiful and such an exotic-looking human that they were taken back to Europe and displayed as though they were magnificent wild animals. The American Indian today is a mere shadow of those ancestors. An anthropologist from the University of California at Berkeley tested Native American Indians and American soldiers in frontier forts and found that the Native Americans were twice as strong as the soldiers.

An anthropologist who visited the Aché tribe of Paraguay was a sub-11-second sprinter in college, yet more than half the adult males in the group could outrun him. This included men he estimated to be in their fifties.

Now, the Aché move through the forest constantly, hunting peccary. They go quietly at a brisk walk or sometimes jog and then sprint after their prey when it is close at hand. They consume roughly 5,000 calories daily – a huge amount, but they need all that energy to keep going. We require less than half that to get through our sedentary days.

Physically and genetically, we are built to run fast and climb trees easily. But few of us over the age of eleven do so. Which is why we're now at the gym.

*

After the bike I head for the leg machines. Because the hamstring muscles – the biceps femoris – are so large, working them first keeps my body temperature up and thereby tells the pituitary to keep pumping out growth hormone.

First stop is the leg curl. This one requires you to lie on your belly and lift the weight behind your ankles. There are also seated versions that make you push the weight down.

Most people here choose a suitable weight and then do two or three sets of eight to ten repetitions, with a minute's break between sets. Instead, I build my sets in a hierarchy, like this: First, fifteen repetitions using a relatively light weight, which I move slowly. That starts the burn, which is the sign I'm looking for. Then, I get up, add more weight – maybe a third of what was on there – and, without taking a break, do eight reps, a little more quickly than the first. Finally, I add still more weight, up around my maximum, and do four reps, quickly. And that's that.

There's a good reason for this hierarchy of repetitions and weight levels. It matches the sequence in which your three main types of muscle fibres go to work. The slow-twitch fibres go first – they exhaust themselves on the first set, with light weight and a high number of reps. The slow-twitch fibres primarily burn fat. On the second set, they recruit the intermediate-twitch muscles for assistance – and they, too, are used up. Those muscles burn both glycogen and fat. You need to push through slow- and intermediate-twitch fibres first in order to summon the grade-A stuff: the fast-twitch fibres. They go to work on the final, heaviest set. They are the ones you want to mobilise, since they burn glycogen now and later, during recovery, fat – in fact, they burn eight times as much energy as the slow-twitch fibres. They are also the most valuable muscle fibres when it comes to strength and body composition. Essentially, to be strong means to have plenty of fast-twitch muscle fibre.

The conventional wisdom requires you to wait a minute or even more between sets – 'recovery time', as it is called. This, too, is wrong-headed in my opinion. There's no advantage in letting the muscle recover too much; the point here is to work it hard. You want to burn off the blood sugar contained in your muscles as quickly as you can, and you need intense work to do that.

Once the glycogen is gone, the lactic acid floods in. That's what causes the burn. That painful sensation tells me that my body has shifted from using glucose as energy to using fat. That shift is crucial. The burn is your body's way of protecting the muscles – lactic acid exhausts the muscle and makes it impossible to continue. Without that safety mechanism in place, you could work the muscle tissue until it is destroyed.

However, I do *not* perform an exercise 'to failure', meaning the point at which I literally am unable to do another repetition. For a number of reasons, pushing a muscle to where it can do no more is a bad idea.

First, doing that probably means you are struggling through the last reps, breaking proper form, gritting your teeth, potentially injuring a tendon or joint as you try hero-ically to reach the point of total muscle exhaustion. It's unnecessary, and all that grunting is ugly on the ears.

Another reason I don't like the idea of working a muscle to failure is that you are here at the gym to seek success, and the brain records every failure as exactly that: you failed. It's a bad habit, especially in pursuit of health.

After working the hamstrings, I go directly to the seated leg-extension machine to balance out the movement I've just done. This exercise works the front of the thigh. Again, I do this in the 15–8–4 rep sequence, adding weight and speed with each set.

The final stop for the lower-body workout is the leg press. There are several kinds, but the seated one is best because it puts less stress on your back. This is also superior, for the same reason, to doing squats with a heavy barbell resting on your shoulders. But the action is essentially the same, to use both feet to push away a heavy load. This is a good measure of strength – men in good shape can move at least double their body weight in this exercise, women a little less.

I will often perform a variation on this by using both legs to push the weight out but just one to lower it. It's called a 'negative' because most of the exertion is in the lowering, not the lifting. In every exercise, you can usually move about 40 per cent more in the negative part of the movement than in the 'positive', or lifting phase, where you work against gravity. Lowering presents its own challenge because you're not fighting against gravity, you're trying to stop it.

A negative, in any exercise, is a great muscle-builder. It actually tears the fibres, which isn't as bad as it sounds – they then grow back larger and stronger than before. It's also called an 'eccentric movement'. It is extremely taxing and should be done with care. Later in this chapter, in the section on advanced exercising, I will describe the occasional workouts I do of nearly all negatives.

Now we're through with legs, it's time to move along to the upper-body workout.

My upper-body training routine also starts with the biggest muscles, to keep the growth hormone flowing and the heart pumping. So we'll begin with the back. There are many ways to work those muscles, but I'm going to begin with a seated cable row, in a hierarchical 15–8–4 set. To balance that, I move next to a barbell row done in a steep, almost standing position rather than the usual bent-over pose, so I work the upper trapezius from a new angle – more neck and shoulder muscles being recruited now. I won't do many of these because I don't want to tax my cervical vertebrae. This is more of a finishing move than anything else, done to improve symmetry of the trunk.

A word here about the concept of symmetry. Having a well-balanced figure seems more a cosmetic concern than anything else, but it's not. There are some exercises I do only for symmetry's sake. You will notice that I don't do an exercise that nearly everybody in the gym does routinely – bicep curls. For weight trainers, biceps are an obsession. They are 'mirror muscles' – guys love working on their arms because they respond well to weight training and make an impressive show when you stare at yourself in the mirror.

But the fact is that many of the upper-body exercises you'll do already work the biceps and triceps, the muscle on the back of the upper arm. And face it, in the course of your daily life, how much arm power do you really need? I do curls or work the triceps only when I look at myself and see an imbalance.

That symmetry should be everywhere – upper body to lower, front of limb to back. Males and females alike should be shaped like an X: broader at the shoulders and hips, narrow at the waist. From an evolutionary perspective, symmetry is a reliable indication of health. In children, developmental diseases result in gross body asymmetry.

For our purposes, being in symmetry means you're probably in good shape. It shows you've attained balance in movement and in muscle groups, so there is less chance of injury while working out.

After the barbell row exercise, I move on to the chest workout, specifically the upper part of the pectoral muscles, just under your collarbone, which is where you need strength most. I find that weightlifters devote too much effort to building a massive chest, especially with the bench press exercise. You don't need all that bulk. And it looks grotesque. Here I will do an incline dumbbell press, sitting on a bench at a 45-degree angle, and using dumbbells so each side of my body works individually.

Shoulders are important, but you've been working them all along in your upper-body exercises, so I have just one routine left to do, the lateral raise machine, which works the deltoids (the muscles at the very top of your arm). This is more a finishing move than anything else, and I'll do it at one of those side-lift machines. You don't want to punish the shoulder muscles too much since they are prone to injury. Some days I'll do this as a negative exercise – I'll raise the weights with both arms but then lower with just one.

I tend not to spend much time working abdominal muscles as such. Whether you feel it or not, we've been working the abs all along. That's because we do the abdominal brace in every exercise. This means we lightly contract the abdominal muscles and maintain proper curvature of the lower back at all times, to develop a kind of postural strength. Posture is a full-time event. And the most fatigue resistant muscles you have – your abs and your spinal erectors – must be engaged in maintaining proper posture.

We will actually do an abdominal exercise – but only one, an ab curl. We make this quite intense by pre-contracting the abdominal muscles before we begin the exercise. The curl is done by lying flat on the floor or an elevated bench, bending the knees and placing the feet flat, just under the hips. Once in this position, the upper trunk is raised from the pelvis to lift the shoulders. I imagine that I am pressing some object in front of me upwards by holding my arms out and curling with the abdominal muscles. You can even increase the resistance by having someone resist the upward push in the arms and hands.

This exercise can be done from side to side as well as upwards. By doing this, the intercostal muscles in the ribcage are strengthened. A six-pack will appear if and when the fat underneath the skin in the abdominal region becomes thin enough.

Finally, whenever I walk I focus on maintaining the abdominal brace posture. If you do this, the muscles will become very strong and you will have all the size you might want. But keep in mind that having large abdominal muscles is not desirable. They only look good when they are contracted.

That's the workout. We're through.

Some women, in particular, won't even try weight training. They fear it will turn them thick and bulky. But lifting weights is even more important for women than for men.

First, women need to preserve their skeletal mass if they want to avoid osteoporosis. And building muscle mass is a crucial component. It's a commonplace occurrence now – an elderly person falls and breaks a hip, rendering him or her permanently unable to walk. My mother broke both of hers and was never the same. She underwent surgery to fix it, but hip operations involve a large loss of blood flow and seem to affect mental acuity.

Even better than surviving a fall, of course, is preventing one. And the best way to do that is to have sufficient muscle mass, especially the fast-twitch kind, to keep you upright. Women tend to have less of that than men, which is why they need to do more to maintain it.

It's true for women (as for men) that putting your muscle under the acute stress of a weight-lifting session releases growth hormone, which does *not* make you look like a bodybuilder. But it does stimulate fat burning and increase your sensitivity to insulin, which stops your body from storing more fat in the future.

Women do not have sufficient testosterone to build serious muscle mass even if they wanted to. For that you'd need to inject testosterone or a related steroid. Working out with weights won't make you big – just strong.

*

I've taken you along on a typical workout at the gym. But, as I've said repeatedly in this book, variety and randomness and intermittency are vital when it comes to maintaining good health in human beings. So there's really no such thing as a typical day at the gym for me. I've been doing my best to avoid dictating how you should structure your workouts. Giving you a routine to slavishly follow would defeat my entire purpose.

I actually have several different types of workout I use at the gym. One is the so-called eccentric workout, which uses negative movements. This is an intense way to do it – as I said earlier, it tears the muscle fibres, thus making them grow back stronger and larger. This adaptation can be done for arms, delts, shoulders, chest and legs. The principle is always the same: you can handle more weight in the lowering phase of an exercise than in the lifting. So you use both arms, or legs, to get the weight up, and then just one to set it back down. You need to experiment a little to determine how much weight you can control in the downward phase. *These exercises are best done on weight machines rather than with free weights, for safety's sake.*

Another thing I do is called alactic exercise, meaning a kind that does not cause lactic acid to be released into the muscle. I do just one repetition of an exercise, for five sets. The weight is high, about as much as I am able to lift for that single rep. This is a hard workout too, not for beginners. You have to be careful or you'll get hurt. But it builds a huge amount of strength in a short time.

In any event, we're finished at the gym. Now is the time that lots of people feel free to reward themselves with a hearty meal for having worked out so hard. But that's a bad idea.

It is only after the workout is done that the fat-burning actually begins. And this is why you shouldn't eat anything right before or after exercise. Eating shuts down the fat-burning phase. Replenishing the glycogen in the muscle with one of those sports drinks that contain so much sugar along with the electrolytes also shuts down the growth hormone and leads to the release of insulin, all of which are counterproductive. A good workout elevates your insulin sensitivity for up to ten hours, affording ample time for the entry of nutrients, including protein and glycogen, into the muscle.

Eating right after a workout also suppresses gene expression. If you go to the gym hungry and stay that way for an hour after you're through, you are burning more fat, improving your hormonal state, and therefore taking maximum advantage of all that hard work.

Exercise actually offsets the effect of the so-called obesity gene. It increases your insulin sensitivity, it burns fat and increases your store of lean muscle tissue. That ratio must be maintained in the correct zone – roughly 11 per cent body fat for males, 18 per cent for females – if you are going to have a shot at a vital old age. Losing fat and gaining muscle may actually increase your weight, since muscle is denser than fat and weightier, too. This is why measures such as weight or Body Mass Index, while important, are totally secondary to body composition.

The main thing to remember is that exercise is not simply something you do to help you lose weight. It is a crucial component of how your body adapts to its environment, and it is absolutely necessary for good health. If you don't do it you are depriving the human organism of something as vital as food, water and sunlight.

Also, there is the not insignificant fact that exercise, if done properly, will make you more beautiful. It will maintain your body in the shape it was meant to take, meaning having shoulders and hips larger than your waist (but not by much), whether you are male or female, and no protruding belly, with your form as sleek and graceful as nature intended, skeleton and muscles evident (though not *too* evident), articulating your limbs and torso. We tell one another not to judge a book by its cover, but the truth is that a great deal can be determined about your health just by looking at you. Strong muscles unobstructed by excess fat, good posture, taut skin, colour that is neither too pale nor too ruddy (a sure sign of inflammation), overall proper proportions, a general air of wellbeing – these are the signs we all recognise, instinctively, as being evidence of good health. You didn't need an expert to tell you that.

interlude
Death by Exercise

I keep a file entitled 'Death by Exercise', a collection of stories about marathoners and other long-distance runners who have died while working out. I am convinced of the connection between excessive aerobic exercise and ill health.

A friend of mine, a retired marine, had a heart attack on a long bicycle training ride as he prepared for an upcoming triathlon. I wrote about him on my blog:

I think our marines are about as tough and brave as any-one can be. Our Community Manager is a retired marine. When I first saw him about two years ago, he was tan and lean and had a shaved head. He looked terrific; erect and leather tough.

What happened to him, I wondered, when he came by my house last week. He was pale, kind of softish, with too much tissue hanging out everywhere, and limping. I asked him why. He pulled or tore a hamstring doing a 10K. This is his third tear in two years.

I knew he had been doing triathlons for the past two years, but I hadn't seen him up close for some time. I was sad and surprised to see how he looked.

The tan is gone because he trains indoors, riding the stationary bike, logging miles on the treadmill, and swimming laps in the indoor pool. The hamstring tears have been nagging because he won't stop training or doing events. So, he has a more or less constant limp.

Why did be become fatter when he was exercising so much? He eats the kind of junk runners have been taught to rely on. He does all the carbo-load meals preceding each event. (Does anybody still believe loading works? Apparently, but the belief is bogus. Only a depleted muscle from over-training requires anything like a load. And the CHO (carbohydrate) load ramps up insulin, blood sugar and stress hormones.) He eats every kind of CHO you can lay your hands on; potato crisps are consumed in large quantities. He may permanently damage his hypothalamus-pituitary-adrenal axis.

Why go through all this pain and misery? Well, marines are tough and he has made a commitment to do the triathlons. He now is known in the community as a participant and takes pride in it, even though it has made him less healthy and effective. And not so tough-looking any more.

We are made more for walking and sprinting than for jogging. The fact is, few hunters ever literally ran down prey over the long distance of a marathon. Native Americans could bring down a horse in a matter of a few days, but that was done primarily by spooking the animal and then trailing it at a distance. We sometimes needed to sprint at the decisive moment, when closing in for the kill, although human ingenuity commonly worked better, as when hunters would drive their prey into traps or dead ends from which they could not escape. We definitely needed to sprint when we ourselves were the prey. Beyond that, however, hunters lived by the sensible maxim that led our ancestors to exert no more effort than was absolutely necessary.

As in all exercise, intermittency and variety are the goals in aerobic workouts. You want to stop and start, go in an instant from walking to running at top speed for forty or fifty yards, then amble along until the urge to sprint overtakes you again. When you do this, you exercise all the different types of muscle fibre, whereas joggers work only the slow- and intermediate-twitch kinds. Jogging also wastes time because you need to do it for long periods to see any benefit. Mixing up sprints with walks is safer for your heart, too. And there's less stress on your knees, ankles, hips, feet and back.

You are getting a good cardio workout just by lifting weights as I suggest, without much of a break between sets or stations. Your heart should be pumping and your lungs working when you do it vigorously and with a sense of purpose. If you still feel the need for more aerobic exercise, find a game to play. Tennis, squash and rollerblading, for instance, are intense, stop-and-start activities, meaning they burn all three kinds of muscle fibre. And they have the added advantage of being fun.

Lately I've been playing a lot of tennis, maybe four times a week, which is all the running I need. When I do my sprints, I'll go once a week to a nearby field and race forty yards, then stop, and repeat this a few times. If I lived near the beach I'd go a couple of times a week and do my sprints on the dry, loose sand, not the wet, packed part. Then I'd take a leisurely stroll for 45 minutes or so. Sprinting first releases growth hormone, and so the body goes on burning fat as you walk afterwards.

Here's another great aerobic workout: Simply jump as high as you can, and land in a squat with your thighs parallel to the ground. Do a dozen of those in rapid succession and see how you feel.

I always take a twenty-minute walk after dinner, no matter where I am, not to burn energy but for the pleasure of it. Whenever I travel, I walk constantly, climb stairs when possible, and take my rollerblades when I can. It's my way of exercising away from home.

If you enjoy it, basketball is a great game from the aerobic perspective, with constant moving, sprinting, stopping on a dime, jumping and diving. Look at the physiques of professional athletes – none of them look as powerful as basketball players. They test as the leanest of all pros, around 8 per cent body fat. Only NFL defensive backs and running backs come close. They, too, move in unpredictable, varied ways – jogging one second, running full-tilt the next, cutting and swerving.

If you need more proof, go to an athletics meeting, then tell me: would you rather look like the milers or the sprinters? The distance runners are stringy, emaciated, haunted. The sprinters look like classical Greek statuary. Keep in mind that the first person to run a marathon, Pheidippides, collapsed and died at the finish line. Marathoners actually have suppressed immune systems. As I'm writing this, I read that three runners just dropped dead during the Detroit marathon – one of them a 26-year-old man, another just 36, both in good health, or so they thought.

Finally, the fact that too much aerobic exercise causes harmful oxidation should also be taken as a sign that, from an evolutionary perspective, our bodies are not well adapted to jogging. The mortality curve is J-shaped: it declines with exercise, hits a bottom, and then rises. The over-exercised fare no better than the under-exercised.

Walking and sprinting are the safest and most beneficial forms of aerobic exercise. Perhaps not coincidentally, they are also the most enjoyable. A sprint is exhilarating, child-like fun. It brings a taste of animalistic wildness and abandon to your workouts. And I shouldn't have to explain the pleasures of a nice, brisk walk outdoors.

five
my journey

It seems as though I have been researching this book all my life.

I began lifting weights and taking an interest in diet at the age of 14. As I have heard many others say, it all began in a garage with a 90-pound weight set. My gains came quickly so, at 16, I joined a gym operated by John Furbotnik, a former Mr America. John's gym was a hang-out for Olympic athletes from the Pasadena Athletic Club and I wanted to be around them. I weighed 196 pounds at age 16 (almost 60 years later I weigh about the same), and began lifting in the demanding Olympic style because it was more athletic than what I had been doing.

I had hopes of playing professional baseball and felt that the speed and power I developed were what I needed. It was a good move because few ballplayers then lifted weights, and it made me strong and quick. I signed a contract with the Hollywood Stars, a minor league team that was part of the Pittsburgh Pirates organisation, right out of high school. But my eyesight and ambitions got the better of my baseball career. I went on to UCLA, where I got my PhD in economics. After a few years working in think-tanks, I became an academic so I could follow my own interests in research.

My main interest was in what was *not* known in my field, which took me into the realm of complex systems, wild variations and extreme events – the so-called 'black swans' that author Nassim Nicholas Taleb writes about. This led me back to Hollywood, not to play baseball but to study the movie business and how it adapted to uncertainty. I didn't know it at the time, but this was excellent preparation for the study of metabolism. I wrote a book about the economics of Hollywood and settled into the University of California Department of Economics and Institute for Mathematical Behavioral Sciences for the last twenty years of my career.

*

My education in metabolism began the year I was Visiting Scholar at the University of Chicago, during the blizzard of 1979. My youngest son, Brandon, developed type-1 diabetes there, probably from a viral infection that triggered a strong immune response. The doctors believed that my son's pancreas suffered collateral damage from the fire-power his immune system aimed at the virus. When this happens, insulin secretion in the important beta cells of the pancreas stops or is severely depressed.

Only type-1 diabetics suffer this autoimmunity, for reasons that are still unclear. There is a genetic link – my wife Bonnie later developed diabetes, too – but something has to trigger the expression of the genes that cause this excessive response from the immune system. My guess is that both my wife and son had very active and aggressive immune systems, since they almost never got sick. In Brandon's and Bonnie's cases, their immune systems permanently altered their metabolisms.

Because I was an academic at heart, I responded to this crisis by going to the university bookstore. I bought books on diabetes and metabolism and a large textbook on endocrinology that I owned until a few months ago, when I donated it to the local library. I learned as much as I could about insulin and diabetes. Eventually, I knew enough to discuss them intelligently with Brandon's doctors, and even to have friendly arguments with them on treatment and insulin injection doses.

The meals were our most contentious topic. The experts wanted my son to eat cereal or pancakes with syrup and orange juice for breakfast, sandwiches or pasta for lunch with jelly for dessert, and beans or potatoes and low-fat meats for dinner. Carbs were friendly, the doctors maintained, and fat was the enemy. The American Diabetes Association still recommends a high-carb, low-fat diet some thirty years later.

But it was evident to me that my son was eating wrong. He was getting too much carbohydrate, and injecting too much insulin to manage the load it imposed on his damaged metabolism. Each dose of carbohydrate had to be followed by an injection of insulin or his blood glucose would rise too much. But if we injected too much insulin, his glucose level would drop dangerously, and he became jittery and angry. If this condition deepens, it can lead to unconsciousness and death. Brandon would sometimes even refuse to take a glucose tablet, a problem many diabetics experience as their blood glucose drops and they become emotional and stubborn. Their brains, in glucose crisis, descend into primitive regions where the cortex loses control.

As you may know, insulin's job is to extract glucose (a form of sugar) from the bloodstream to store it for later use. But things go wrong when the body receives more of this hormone than it needs. It will actually withhold glucose from the bloodstream even when the brain is being denied this essential fuel and nears unconsciousness. The other hormones that can also mobilise energy are powerless to help. The brain in those instances *could* extract the glucose it needs from elsewhere in the body, mainly the liver – except that the insulin overrides the hormones responsible for that task. Insulin is essential but also potentially dangerous; it is the instrument of choice in movies (and sometimes, in reality) when a doctor wants to murder his or her spouse or a rogue nurse wants to kill patients.

I knew as an economist that it made no sense to try to manage blood glucose, which is a flow, with a storage hormone like insulin. Eating to take in carbohydrate and then hoping to inject just the right amount of insulin to utilise the glucose was a crude, imprecise policy. It was likely to make my son fat, because safety required that he consume more sugar than he needed, lest his brain get too little glucose and go into shock.

Eventually, we got off the carbs-insulin seesaw. But not just yet.

My education in metabolism was furthered when my wife Bonnie also developed type-1 diabetes, twelve years after Brandon. We weren't sure why this happened, and neither were her doctors. My hunch was that she had been taking too much thyroid medicine, which stressed her metabolism to breaking point. We had better tools for diabetics by this point; meters had become simple and inexpensive so we could measure blood glucose more accurately than when Brandon was diagnosed.

Bonnie ate as her doctors suggested because she loved pasta and potatoes and pancakes and bread. But injecting insulin to manage her starchy diet made her gain weight, too, and soon she was doing her best to balance between too little insulin and too much. We went through many a night with her deep in insulin shock as I tried to get some glucose into her. It was a nightmare.

I began to examine Bonnie's testing numbers and correlate her blood glucose with her meals. I used my training in statistics to look for patterns in her readings, to see if I could find reasons behind her worst episodes of insulin shock and high glucose. I tried to see what sorts of foods increased blood glucose and what insulin doses were necessary to bring the levels back to a healthy range.

It soon became apparent that striving to keep blood glucose in a narrow range using insulin injections was counterproductive, even dangerous; this is a connection that research has now established. Both my wife and my son had too many episodes of low blood glucose that put them close to insulin shock. These ordeals were exhausting them. They became depressed and gained weight. Brandon, who had been lean, became a chubby boy. Bonnie, who had been a slim *Vogue* cover girl, put on weight and then dropped it again in cycles. She was still beautiful, but the stress was taking its toll.

We figured out that every deep fall or steep rise in blood glucose made similar events even more likely later. This suggested that the brain has a metabolic memory that records past events and responds in similar ways when they occur again. The brain was learning to make the adjustments necessary to bring blood glucose into a stable range. But soon it was over-reacting, like a driver over-steering as he tries to control a swerving car. The cycling back and forth is itself dangerous. Some type-1 diabetics become what doctors call 'brittle', meaning that they swing too easily from high to low blood glucose levels.

We needed to teach the brain a better strategy. I believed we had to let the brain learn to mobilise glucose from sources *inside* the body instead of relying on external supplies, meaning carbs. We had to use less insulin, and to do that we had to eat fewer foods that raised blood glucose.

The NED developed directly out of our experiments with foods and how Bonnie's bloodstream responded to them. She tested her blood glucose after each meal, and then we looked at the data to see what had elevated that level and how much insulin was needed to bring it back to a healthy range.

Pasta and potatoes sent her blood glucose through the roof, requiring a large injection of insulin to bring it back. So pasta and potatoes were the first entries on our list of offending dishes. We identified all such foods and simply cut them out. We did not just reduce her intake of these foods – we banished them. I did not want her reactivating old metabolic memories by eating small amounts of offending dishes. The list of forbidden foods grew over time, with each meal being an experiment. We did not know it at the time, but twenty-five years ago we were creating our own Glycaemic Index, which is now the basis for the Zone, the South Beach Diet and other popular eating regimens.

Right behind pasta and potatoes, bread made the list of banned foods because they, too, prompted a large rise in blood glucose. Breakfast cereal and cinnamon buns, Bonnie's favourite, went on the list next.

The programme was a success. Soon, a minimal amount of insulin was needed to keep my wife and son stable. One doctor refused to believe Bonnie was a diabetic because she was injecting so little insulin.

Today it is generally accepted that there's a strong link between diabetes and obesity. Overweight people (even non-diabetics) are often insulin-resistant, meaning their bodies don't respond properly to the existing insulin levels, and so they require more of the hormone. An important cause of insulin resistance among type-2 diabetics is the inflammation caused by elevated blood glucose and excess body fat. So you see, fat isn't just this stuff inside that increases your girth. It is metabolically active tissue with organ-like capabilities. Fat secretes hormones that make other tissues resist the action of insulin. An overweight person may require more insulin than a slender person to manage glucose.

The fresh vegetables and fruit we were consuming drastically reduced my wife's inflammation as she lost weight and excess body fat. In response, her insulin sensitivity increased. Best of all, we ate wonderfully on our new diet. We didn't feel the least bit deprived. After a while, it didn't require any self-control, which is a good thing for several reasons. Most people don't realise that acts of self-control are such hard mental work that they actually deplete the glucose levels in the brain. Therefore you will lack willpower when glucose is low or cannot be mobilised effectively. It's a big reason why diets don't work.

Bonnie's past glucose crises began to fade in memory as her stress fell. The neural networks seemed to re-form as the old ones faded for lack of use, so much so that eating any of the offending substances left all of us feeling sick and bloated.

From then on, I cooked dinner quite a lot, which was a new experience for me. Even my eating had to improve: I had been on the relatively high-carbohydrate diet that was making the rounds in athletic circles. I recall seeing pictures of Olympic athletes 'carbing out' before events, eating big plates of pasta. I never ate that way on a daily basis, but before some of my athletic events I would often load up on starches. Now, I had to learn to eat differently.

I would stop at the store on the way home from work and browse the produce section, looking for something fresh and colourful. Next I went to the seafood or meat aisles, and then headed home to make dinner with whatever I had found. My shopping trips were confined to the periphery of the supermarket, meaning I seldom ventured into the centre aisles where the processed and packaged foods were located. I usually cooked more than we would eat, so we could have breakfast, lunch or another dinner from leftovers. It was faster than fast food. Much better and cheaper, too.

*

So this was a breakthrough for us, but it was still just our little family project. Then, one day in my office, I was talking with a graduate student in anthropology who had come in to see me about a topic she was working on. It had something to do with reciprocity between members of a tribe.

We talked about meat sharing and I brought up our new diet. I told her that my family and I had begun eating only fresh vegetables, fruits, nuts, seafood and meat. She told me that the tribal members she studied ate the same way. It should have been obvious to me, but I hadn't thought about it: I had come up with a typical hunter-gatherer meal plan.

Intrigued, I made the rounds among my anthropologist colleagues at the Institute to discuss this and to ask what I should read on the subject. I found it ironic that these people who knew so much about hunter-gatherers all loved pasta and bread. Many of the scholars were overweight. One evolutionary psychologist was downright obese. I thought, if he knows so much about the human mind and its evolution, why is he so fat? I think he had separated his knowledge of science from his personal habits, as many people seem to do, by giving little thought to what they eat.

I read about and discussed the human genome, our library of genes. The modern human genome is about 50,000 to 100,000 years old. Little has changed during that time except for some variation in genes that are localised, population-specific adaptations to disease, and some recent ones that involve nutrition, such as the ability to metabolise the sugar lactose contained in milk.

I began to look into the relationship between the original human diet that was consumed by hunter-gatherers and our genetic make-up. I focused on 40,000 BC, when fully modern humans emerged. The diet they consumed back then was strikingly similar to what my family and I had developed as we attempted to control diabetes.

The current debate over fat versus carbohydrate in the diet is anchored totally in the modern idea of eating. This is really an argument over fads, because virtually every modern diet is just a small variation on bad nutritional thinking. Excellent research has been done by many scholars, notably Loren Cordain, whose *Paleo Diet* book provides guidance.

I came to think of our diet, derived through careful experimentation with the foods that exist today, as a modern form of the original diet. We were not trying to mimic the Palaeolithic Diet, or to 'eat palaeo', as the expression goes. It's not necessary to do anything so drastic. I think our genes can handle contemporary life just fine if we help them with diet and activity. In fact, I believe that the current epidemics of insulin resistance and metabolic disease are really an attempt by our genes to keep us alive and healthy on a diet that misdirects our metabolisms.

Oddly, it was my understanding of decentralised economic systems and their use of price to guide the allocation of resources that led me to address the big question of human metabolism: how does your body know where and when to send energy and nutrients? Inside, you are not a single organism – you are a vast colony of billions of cells bound in a complex dance of co-operation and competition that somehow sustains life. There is no centralised control. Each cell has its genetic programme whose expression is influenced by its neighbours and its development sequence in such a way that one cell can be liver tissue and another can be cardiac muscle.

The cells are specialised, as we say in economics. They perform their individual functions in response to the neural, hormonal and other signals they receive from their surroundings. Good health is possible only if cells follow those signals correctly. Disease, cell damage and many other insults result from miscommunication and destroy the internal order that is required to keep you alive and healthy.

As we've discussed, those genes evolved at a time when humans lived in a world vastly different from today's. We are genetically built to thrive on a 40,000-year-old diet. The farther we stray from that, the more we endanger our health.

But eating was only half of the puzzle. I took my economics analogy further, applying the dynamic statistical models I developed in my research to the movement of wild animals, children at play, sports events. I would eventually use this to understand the complex energy dynamics of Palaeolithic hunter-gatherers as they foraged for food. There were periods of feast and famine and mixtures of physical activity that varied enormously in intensity and duration.

Hunger motivates movement. This is a genetically engineered survival tactic. If you are starving, you have a powerful reason to get up and do something about it. Hunger also alters your bloodstream – it releases adrenaline and growth hormone to mobilise fat as fuel. That's a good moment to exercise, if you're interested in getting maximum results. An experimenter once told me he could not get his lab rats to do their mandatory exercise unless they were hungry. One well-fed rat would just sit on the treadmill and let the wheel rub the fur of its behind.

What was most revealing about trying to model the Palaeolithic energy environment was how our ancestors moved. A hunter had to walk long distances, sprint, and then, in the kill, had to execute abrupt, violent motions. If the hunt were successful, he'd have to lift and haul a heavy load back home. A gatherer, too, walked far depending on what she sought, and then had to return home bearing a burden. Most of life was random and unpredictable. There was no such thing as a 'typical' activity. A hunter expended energy in great bursts of activity and treks of varying length, but then, for a lot of the time, did absolutely nothing.

From that insight, it was a short leap to exercising in a new way. I began doing intermittent, high-intensity work-outs, to emulate what I thought a prehistoric man would have to do in the course of his normal existence. There is now abundant research that shows this kind of workout gets better results than the grinding routine of moderately taxing, hyper-regimented exercise that many trainers still dictate to their clients.

I began to exercise less than ever before, but harder. There was no standard workout routine – I never did the same exercises in the same order twice. I still lifted, pushed, pulled, reached, but as the spirit moved me, not according to some textbook plan. I also varied the time of day I exer-cised, and the amount of time between workouts. I might spend a few minutes in the gym one day, an hour the next time, and then stay away altogether for a day or two, to give myself time to recover. Sometimes I'd just find a field nearby and try to simulate some brief but intense 'fight or flight' moments, as if I were chasing something (or something were chasing me).

It worked splendidly. Already muscular and lean, I hit new levels of both. A famous sculptress asked me to pose for her (I was in my late sixties at the time) and people at the gym started watching my workouts. They asked what I ate and did to look the way I did. They never believed me when I told them, because it went contrary to everything they 'knew' about fitness.

My diet and exercise had altered my metabolism to express my inner hunter-gatherer. I had become a 21st-century caveman.

*

And that was my private journey, which soon became a public one through a suitably 21st-century method: my blog.

That came to be in a somewhat roundabout way. I already had a university website, devoted to my courses and studies in economics and uncertainty. Then, in the early 1990s, I decided to put into writing all I had learned about health, in an essay titled 'Evolutionary Fitness'. I posted it on the site, and then put up more writings on health, diet and fitness, and soon I was getting so many emails on those subjects that I established a blog of my own.

Like Nassim Nicholas Taleb, I had been studying the consequences of extreme events, though my study was confined to the motion-picture industry. I had used his landmark book, *Fooled by Randomness*, in my courses on extreme events beginning in 2002, because there really was nothing else written before on the topic that was readable for an undergraduate student. I responded avidly because of my belief that economics is driven far more by extreme events than by the steady drip of the average.

This view came from my research on motion pictures, but it turns out that extreme events have a huge effect on human metabolism, too. My research had led me to regard life as being far from an equilibrium process. There is now a huge amount of research establishing this point of view very clearly. It does lead to very simple insights about human metabolism and health.

For instance, many of the statistical distributions one finds in the research are far from routine or normal. This means that the average tends to be dominated by extreme variations. So the word 'average' often means nothing when it comes to statistics or measurements, whether of the motion-picture business or of human health. In the latter, the average is rapidly becoming the picture of poor health.

The average level of insulin, for example, has drifted upwards over time, so that to be 'normal' now in this regard is not a good thing. It may just mean you are as unhealthy as your neighbour. The average testosterone level of males has declined over the past two decades. That's another realm where I would rather be abnormal.

The dietary concern for average energy balance, too, is absolutely misplaced, in my opinion. No living creature ever lived in perfect energy balance, where calorie input and output were always exactly equal. The diet experts would have you strive for such a state. But it's a totally unnatural way to live, impossible to maintain, anxiety-causing, and not much fun. Even if you could live that way, it wouldn't make you healthy. How many reasons do you need to abandon this popular form of nonsense?

Initially, the blog was concerned with a variety of topics that grew out of my academic research and my interest in politics and economics. Much to my surprise, traffic grew rather rapidly. I had never advertised or sought out search engines or done any of the hundreds of things people do now in order to draw visitors. The blog seemed to be a self-organising process. New traffic tended to generate still more new traffic, and at times the growth was explosive.

I think it was the brew of topics that I discussed and my rather unusual perspective that attracted readers. I described the blog as a scientist looking at uncertainty, economics, health and fitness – an odd combination. Remarkably, it attracted a substantial number of scientists and researchers in various fields related to economics, finance, health and fitness. I spent little time looking at who was coming to the blog or where links to it could be found. But quite early on

I noticed a number of distinguished research institutions' websites that included links to mine.

My website grew quickly. Month after month there were visitors from 115 different countries. The number of hits was consistently over 2.5 million per month. Just before I made the blog available by subscription only, I reached 3 million hits. I made friends all over the world just by sitting at my computer, writing down my thoughts. I never chose to advertise the blog or to sell advertising or any products on it. It was just pure content supplied only by me.

What sort of material was I putting up? Whatever I felt like. I think that was an important element in the trust I earned. One of my more unusual posts was called 'All You Need to Know about Zen'. It had more than 20,000 hits the day I posted it and continues to be my best-read entry ever. Soon, the health postings began to attract attention. I was written about in the *New Scientist*, one of the best science magazines available. A PBS programme called *Closer to Truth* called to see if I would appear on an episode entitled 'Can You Really Extend Your Life?' I joined a distinguished group: the host, Dr Robert Kuhn; Dr Sherwin Nuland, a Yale professor and bestselling author; Dr French Anderson, one of the early pioneers of gene therapy; and Dr Roy Walford, a pioneering life-extension researcher and author of *The 120-Year Diet*.

To be invited to appear on the show was a pleasant surprise. I think I surprised the other guests, who probably assumed I would be a kook. Who would expect that an economist had anything sensible to say about human biology? But they surrounded me after the taping and we talked extensively about my approach to health and fitness. I think they were surprised when I told them my age; it turned out that I was among the oldest people on the show.

None of the other guests raised my issue, which was this: at the same time they were talking about life extension, we were seeing a progressive *loss* of healthy longevity in the United States. Little or none of the perspective these wise men offered seemed to have reached the rest of the country. If anything, healthy life expectancy was declining, thanks to a terrible diet, lack of exercise and metabolic disease. The height of Americans has actually declined, and our obesity increased, just in the brief interval since the show was broadcast at the start of the century. Our high-minded academic discussion about the possibilities of extending life and improving its quality had little to do with reality.

The host, Dr Kuhn, remarked that merely doing the show was stressful. Apparently it was, because he ate nervously throughout the taping. The spread laid out for the guests included sweet rolls, muffins and other simple carbs, even candy bars. When I told this brilliant man that he was eating so much junk because his insulin was too high, and that mixing insulin with stress hormones caused stress eating, he was taken aback. I disagreed with the diet and exercise advice he promulgated – eat your grains and do your cardio – and told him so. Why emphasise grains, I asked, when they cause insulin resistance, provoke the immune system, damage the gut and contain too many simple carbo-hydrates? He had no answer. Whether his attitude or diet changed, I cannot say, since I lost contact with him. Sadly, my fellow guest Dr Walford, the life-extension guru, did not live to be 120; he died just three years after the show.

My ideas have found a particularly hospitable home in Great Britain, thanks in part to a newspaper story that was carried about me in *The Times*. In it, the writer Bryan Appleyard described me in a way that has stuck, to my bemusement: he said I look 'like Superman's father'. In London there is even a group that has formed independently, made up of people who follow my philosophy. They had their first meeting in the autumn of 2009 and planned to get together regularly to discuss the programme and swap stories about how it has changed their lives.

I am very happy with my blog now as a private site, available only to subscribers, and plan to keep it that way. No ads get in the way and all the content is my own, expressed in my own way. No hype or miracles, just advice based on science and many years of experience. Throw in the libertarian point of view and the need for freedom and personal expression and you have what my readers seem to crave.

interlude
men, consider this

It has been reported in recent years that testosterone levels in men are mysteriously dropping. During that same period, the epidemic of obesity has been in the news non-stop. It's not a coincidence. It amazes me that so few experts have made a connection between the poor diet of young men and declining levels of the essential male hormone.

You'd think the guys might be a little worried. They should be. The modern diet is feminizing men.

Watch any televised sport and you'll see a big reason it's happening: every edible product being advertised has been found to suppress production of testosterone and increase levels of oestrogen in males: pizza, beer, fast-food burgers and fries, doughnuts and other sweets, fizzy drinks, the so-called 'sports drinks' ... even the protein supplements being sold as aids to muscle building. Each of these foods or supplements produce elevated sugar in the bloodstream which reduces testosterone and increases obesity, which in turn reduces testosterone. Taken all together, this sugar dosing is a massive hit to our masculinity.*

Testosterone is important even beyond the obvious reason that it fuels our sex drive and is, in essence, what makes us male. Insufficient testosterone has been linked with increased risk of death, obesity, type-2 diabetes, heart disease and low sperm count. Women need it, too.

'Both the incidence of low testosterone, or hypo-gonadism, in men and the annual number of testosterone prescriptions are increasing, likely as a result of the obesity epidemic and our aging population,' said Frances Hayes MD, an endocrinologist who recently studied the connection between sugar consumption and hormones. That word, *hypogonadism*, should scare you. It means that getting fat may shrink your testicles, decrease your testosterone and make you less male.†

---

* Alcohol is a prime contributor to hypogonadism and feminization of males, Gordon and Southren. Hypogonadism and feminization in the male: a triple effect of alcohol. 'Alcoholism: Clinical and Experimental Research' (2008) vol. 3. Glucose is almost as bad. Frances Hayes, MD, an endocrinologist at St Vincent's University Hospital in Dublin, Ireland, examined the effect of glucose on testosterone levelsin men. The researchers found that a glucose solution decreased blood levels of testosterone by as much as 25 percent, regardless of whether the men had diabetes, pre-diabetes or normal glucose tolerance.

† The secular decline in testosterone among males is examined in Andersson et al. Secular Decline in Male Testosterone and Sex Hormone Binding Globulin Serum Levels in Danish Population Surveys. Testosterone level is a better predictor than leptin of mortality in aged males, Simon et al. Serum testosterone but not leptin predicts mortality in elderly men. Research Letters: Aging (2009). See Michael Zitzmann. Testosterone deficiency, insulin resistance and the metabolic syndrome, Nature Reviews Endocrinology 5, 673–681 (1 December 2009).

The culprits are all the usual nutritional offenders. Sugar has been found in the lab to lower testosterone. The authors of one scientific study found that a drink of glucose solution decreased blood levels of testosterone by as much as 25 per cent, regardless of whether the men had diabetes or pre-diabetes. Free radicals induced by sugar consumption may also have a hand in lowering testosterone.

Grain-based foods, because they add to our fat stores, also depress testosterone levels. High insulin and low testosterone tend to go together.

Body fat plays an interesting role, too – it actually converts testosterone into oestrogen, the female hormone. The process is called 'aromatising'.

Women need testosterone and men need oestrogen, but when the level gets too high we run into trouble. It's not just being fat that causes some men to develop womanly breasts – it's the overload of female hormones due to bad diet. There are obese men walking around with less testosterone and more oestrogen than their wives.

What about sports drinks? Totally unnecessary. They contain not just too much sugar but too much salt as well. Some people who drink them may begin to retain water. And those protein supplements that supposedly help build muscle often contain as many calories of carbohydrate and sugar as three pieces of pie.

Young men today get too many of their daily calories from alcohol. I've seen studies that say college-age men get as much as one-quarter of their calories from drinking. Alcohol itself lowers testosterone, but it goes beyond that. The ethanol causes the same spike in blood glucose and insulin resistance as any empty calories. The usual bad cascade results – alcohol promotes the storage of fat, and then the fat changes the testosterone into oestrogen. When the body is lacking vitamin A and other nutrients, there is nothing to block or limit this conversion.

Additionally, too much alcohol suppresses appetite; alcoholics tend to be malnourished. A while back there was a proposal to add vitamins to alcoholic drinks for this very reason, but the do-gooders nixed it on the grounds that it might encourage more drinking.

Finally, alcohol promotes inflammation, which worsens insulin resistance. Ethanol is toxic to all the nerves in the body. So, in addition to losing their masculinity, heavy drinkers lose their brains, too.

SiX
underpinnings

First came my boyhood passion for sports and strength.
Next was my immersion in the world of nutritional science
and metabolism because of my wife's and son's diabetes.
And there is also a third element that connects all the dots
and accounts for my fascination with the subject of this
book: the ways in which it has intersected with my intellectual life.

A little background. A great deal of my work as an
economist has been in the study of complex systems, such
as how natural gas prices are determined by the market-
place throughout North America. Not surprisingly, given
that I had grown up in southern California and taught at
a university there, I eventually turned my attention to a
notoriously murky, seemingly impossible to forecast industry: Hollywood.

Since its inception, the people running the motion-
picture business have tried to unlock the mystery of which
decisions lead to financial success and which to failure. At

some point, all the wisdom had been boiled down to this rueful admission by screenwriter William Goldman: 'Nobody knows anything.' That's exactly the kind of axiom that an economist cannot let stand untested. And so in 1995 we gathered box-office revenue data on 300 Hollywood films and began to investigate what separated the winners from the losers.

Our research produced a book and several scholarly papers, the gist of which was this: Goldman was right. There is no way at the outset to plan a movie's success. Neither the choice of stars or directors or writers, nor the genre of movie or the subject matter, were found to make a reliable difference in how the films performed. Some big-budget movies soared at the box office, and others tanked. Small, 'quality' movies made for modest sums exhibited the same range of possibilities (although with smaller stakes, of course). Neither did critical acclaim or scorn seem to matter.

Unlike other industrial products – patio furniture, say, or breakfast cereal – each movie was a unique entity. The exact combination of film, audience and moment in time created a once-only event. The sole predictive factor was how the movie had done thus far: popular movies tended to grow in popularity, as positive word of mouth attracted more filmgoers to the cinema. Unpopular films fell into even deeper disfavour among audiences, and their receipts decreased.

In our attempts to explain the motion-picture business, we even drew on a study Albert Einstein did in the 1920s to try and predict how gas molecules would bounce around and eventually form clusters. He found it impossible to predict where exactly the molecules would gather, but he knew that they would. Similarly, we knew that some movies would succeed and others would not. But that's all we knew. The businesspeople could take advantage of the dynamics of success only by putting their resources behind the winners and cutting their losses on the losers. Simply knowing what they can and cannot control should be valuable information to the studio executives and producers, although in the years since our studies came out it is difficult to see what advantage, if any, the industry has taken of this knowledge.

Meanwhile, my ad hoc study of health, nutrition and fitness continued to deepen. I had already begun to see how looking back at life 40,000 years ago could teach us how to live today. Now I was also beginning to perceive the full complexity of the systems and dynamics that determine whether or not we will be healthy.

At some point I realised the key point: a human being is just another economic system. Indeed, your body contains an entire economy. There is the allocation of assets according to a hierarchy of needs. There are competing interests that sometimes struggle over resources and at other times co-operate for the common good. There are surpluses. There are shortages. Like economies – like the movie industry – your body is a complex, decentralised system poised between chaos and order, a constantly changing situation that is, second by second, atom by atom, also adapting to those changes.

All this ran counter to the popular illusion that what happens inside our bodies is a stable, linear, orderly process controlled by the head office – the brain – which dictates the proper actions of everything below. Far from it. You are made up of electrical, chemical and mechanical components all under the influence of regulatory processes that try to establish equilibrium but never quite succeed. Your pancreatic cells don't take orders from your brain, your blood, or anything else except the DNA that created them. And the same is true for all the billions of cells inside you.

In the movie business, word of mouth reviews, more than anything, were what prompted fans to see one film instead of another, or no film at all. It is a powerful feedback loop made up of millions of small parts, each acting independently. This system has grown exponentially since the advent of the internet. Where once millions of moviegoers chattered, now there are billions, perpetually in contact with one another, weighing in, arguing, linking, connecting and disconnecting, uploading and downloading.

It mimics perfectly what goes on inside our bodies: billions of cells all connected but working autonomously, with no central authority to guide them, taking in information (in the form of nutrients, hormones and so on), reacting, then talking back and forth at the speed of electrons, each one responding in small ways that collectively add up to a powerful force.

'Information cascade' is a term from economics to describe how even a small piece of knowledge can be amplified as it spreads from one decision-maker to another. Your body is also controlled by cascades of information – your bloodstream is hit with a dose of carbs, which is the signal for your pancreas to release insulin, which turns off fat-burning and silences the signal from leptin, the hormone that would ordinarily tell your body that it has adequate reserves of energy and need not store any more.

Likewise, in the ageing cascade we lose metabolic fitness, and as a result insulin rises and we grow more acidic, which further decreases metabolic health, and each event amplifies the momentum of what came before.

Hollywood wanted to believe that there was some stable, easy-to-predict dynamic that ruled the movie business. If there were, decisions could be made and investments taken with confidence in their outcome.

Similarly, health experts used over-simplified analogies – automobile engines and furnaces are two that come to mind – to predict how your metabolism will manage nutrition and weight. All you have to do is burn more fuel than you take in, we were instructed, and you will reliably lose weight. Burn precisely as much as you consume and you will maintain weight. Burn less and you'll gain weight. Simple arithmetic.

This was more a failing of human imagination than anything else. We all like to have things orderly instead of chaotic, to make simple sense of what otherwise seems overwhelmingly complicated. In any event, we now all know how infinitely more complex than a car engine or a furnace your metabolism truly is.

I found myself using concepts from other scientific disciplines to help me understand and explain the human body's workings. Certainly, it is possible to get the practical benefits of Evolutionary Fitness without getting into such esoteric territory. But I found that it helped me, a layman, to engage with the material, to frame what I was learning and express it.

For instance, at around the time of our movie industry studies, chaos theory was becoming fashionable in the sciences. The theory itself was a mathematical concept first trotted out in the nineteenth century, although mathematicians don't understand the word the same way as everybody else does. 'Chaos' theory simply said that certain systems that seem to be random in fact are not – it's just difficult for us to perceive, at the outset, all the subtle factors that set the course and determine the outcome.

In time, chaos theory was being applied in other sciences as well, everything from earthquake science to economics. I found that it helped me to understand how our bodies function, too.

One landmark of chaos theory is the so-called Butterfly Effect. This says that even a very small, unseen occurrence in a far-off place can have a large eventual impact – that if a butterfly flaps its wings in Hong Kong, the resulting breeze can trigger a cascade of atmospheric events and cause a hurricane in Brazil.

This could be used to explain many of the workings of our bodies. Here's a simple one. If you go to the gym on an empty stomach, your body will quickly burn through whatever glycogen is in your muscles and then move on to burning fat, which is the desirable state. But if on your way to the gym you have a sports drink, one with lots of carbs, you will need to burn off the sugars from the drink first. And depending on your workout, you might never get around to burning fat at all. Same exact exercise routine, very different outcomes, all because of your choice of pre-exercise beverage.

Another scientific concept, that of the power law, also comes up often in my discussions of health and fitness.

It is based on the Pareto Principle, named for Italian economist Vilfredo Pareto, who devised it. In essence, it describes the relationship between how common a factor is and how much influence it exerts. It says that the most unusual events will have the greatest impact. Pareto's study, done about a century ago, determined that 80 per cent of privately held land in Italy was owned by 20 per cent of the population (the principle is also called the 80/20 rule, or the law of the vital few). Similar power laws exist all around us.

For instance, in our study of the movie business, we learned that 90 per cent of profits came from 10 per cent of movies. And for directors, 40 per cent of their lifetime revenues will come from a single film. Scientists have found that 40 per cent of a decade's damage due to flood will come from just one flood. The Richter law of earthquakes says that the most common quakes are small, and the rare big ones do nearly all the damage. This relationship between low frequency and high impact is found again and again, in various fields of science, business and elsewhere.

Even in our everyday lives we see power laws. A man will meet many women, for instance, but only a very few – his wife (or wives, as the case may be) – will have a lasting effect on his life. You may work alongside many colleagues, but only a handful will have a significant impact on your career. It is the few memorable moments that count more than the drip-drip of quotidian events.

There is a power law of exercise, too: your least frequent, most extreme exertions will have the greatest influence on your fitness. The peak moments of a workout count for more than the amount of time you spend working out. This is why a series of 40-yard sprints at full speed benefits you more than half an hour of jogging. Or why lifting a weight heavy enough to make your heart pound and your muscles burn counts more than spending hours at the gym always in your comfort zone, never truly challenging your body. When a workout becomes an unvarying, monotonous routine, it loses its effectiveness.

Power law teaches us that the average can be meaningless and even misleading. In the movie business, many films lose money and a few are huge hits, but if you compute the average you may be fooled into thinking that all films earn money – which is far from the case. In fact, it is likely that *no* film earned the average sum.

Similarly, my average output of energy per week may look fairly modest. But the stretches of indolence are offset by two or three sessions of extremely intense activity, which do most to determine my wellbeing. Ancient hunter-gatherers spent much of their time doing little or nothing. And then, every so often, they took action that would exhaust any 21st-century gym rat. Overall, they burned twice as much energy as we do. Lions sleep most of the time. But then they make up for it by chasing down, killing and carrying away an adult gazelle. The lion doesn't try to maintain a steady output of moderate energy. It knows better.

There are people at my gym who waste hours on tread-mills and stairmasters, trudging away but never really pushing themselves to intensity. By doing the same cardio workout day after day, their bodies adapt to that exact level of energy demand but nothing greater. The internal message these people send is that they don't need much fast-twitch muscle fibre, and so it atrophies, and as a result they lose bone mass, too. They remind me of a marathoner who played on my softball team – he could run all day long, but was incapable of beating the throw to first base.

There are other terms and concepts I use that are not normally found in fitness books. Stochasticity, for instance, which is a Greek word meaning randomness or chance. A living human leaves a 'trail' of events and accomplishments that is so complex that it appears to be random. That means there is no model that can compress the information that is required to describe a lifetime. The appearance of random-ness is an acknowledgment of the limits of our knowledge. So it is in markets and in life.

Or fractals, another term from mathematics that refers to jagged lines, such as is found in an electrocardiogram. The heart has no standard beat; it is constantly being acted upon by whatever is going on within and also outside your body. And so the rhythm of the beat varies constantly. If it becomes too random it's a problem, but it's also unhealthy if your heartbeat is too regular and metronomic. The jagged, fractal variations are evidence of your system's adaptability – your heart's ability to respond properly to stimulus. A heart that beats to a fractal pattern follows a power law distribution of the intervals between beats.

My particular form of engagement with the subject of health and fitness has even proven to have a metaphysical side. Evolutionary Fitness has shown me that each of us has what I call an ensemble of stochastic life paths – the choices that we make. You make each choice in life based on your understanding of the possibility that it will take you where you want to be. But you don't determine the outcome, only the probabilities. Each path leads to more choices: a cascade to echo all the other cascades that rule our lives. Choosing the path is the extent of your control – beyond that, it's out of your hands. You choose, and then life rolls the dice.

For example, you can determine what you eat and drink and how you will exercise. But then your genes express themselves as they will. They are beyond your control. You can't even completely determine your genes' environment, since outside factors such as air and water quality, and internal ones like emotional stress, also have a say. I learned about the limits of control when caring for my first wife through her terminal illness. I learned it again in my studies of the movie industry, and now in the course of my ongoing education in EF.

It has even allowed me to recognise, in this thought, the Zen of Evolutionary Fitness: 'There is no failure, only feedback.'

interlude
the Dangers of a
High-Carb Diet

In the *Daily Telegraph* (May 2005), Elizabeth Grice colour-fully described five-time Olympic rowing champion Sir Steven Redgrave's diet and training regime:

Steve Redgrave's description of the body fuel he needed to get him through four training sessions a day in the run-up to his fifth consecutive Olympic gold medal is Bunterish in its amplitude, the drooling dream of any pudding-loving member of the human race who has ever grappled with a weight problem.

To keep up the phenomenal energy levels required for a typical day ploughing the water, Sir Steven needed to consume 6,000 calories, starting with a hefty four Weetabix for breakfast. Between the first two sessions on the Thames, he would down a bowl of porridge, liberally dressed with sugar, or scrambled eggs on toast and a large jug of fruit juice.

Refuelling between the afternoon sessions usually meant soup, followed by a large pasta dish, pudding and another flagon of juice. Back home to toast or malted loaf – even if on the way he may have stopped for petrol and picked up a chocolate bar, a packet of wine gums and a bag of dough-nuts to keep his blood sugar levels up.

For the main meal of the day, spaghetti bolognese would ideally be followed by rice pudding or apple pie and ice cream. A bowl of cereal at bedtime and he would know he had done his bit for England. Arise, if possible, Sir Steve.

Multi-gold medallist swimmer Michael Phelps reportedly consumes 12,000 calories a day, twice as many calories as Steve Redgrave did. Clemente Lisi describes Phelps's diet in the *New York Post* web page (13 August 2008) in the following way:

Phelps' diet – which involves ingesting 4,000 calories every time he sits down for a meal – resembles that of a reckless overeater rather than an Olympian.

Phelps lends a new spin to the phrase 'Breakfast of Champions' by starting off his day by eating three fried-egg sandwiches loaded with cheese, lettuce, tomatoes, fried onions and mayonnaise.

He follows that up with two cups of coffee, a five-egg omelet, a bowl of grits, three slices of French toast topped with powdered sugar and three chocolate-chip pancakes.

At lunch, Phelps gobbles up a pound of enriched pasta and two large ham and cheese sandwiches slathered with mayo on white bread – capping off the meal by chugging about 1,000 calories' worth of energy drinks.

For dinner, Phelps really loads up on the carbs – what he needs to give him plenty of energy for his five-hours-a-day, six-days-a-week regimen – with a pound of pasta and an entire pizza.

He washes all that down with another 1,000 calories' worth of energy drinks.

The caloric intake is fine, given his energy expenditure. He has to consume digestible foods if his stomach is to hold up to the load. So things like pancakes are almost essential.

Note that both reporters adhere to the fallacious 'energy balance' model. They argue that these athletes were protected from obesity because their energy expenditures equalled their intakes. This is not necessarily so.

Athletes who consume large amounts of energy are making tremendous demands on the pancreas. The beta cells of the pancreas that sense and release insulin in response to glucose, and the insulin receptors that respond to insulin, may wear out from repeated assaults of glucose and free radicals. Inflammation attacks and makes the cells and cell receptors less sensitive. Consequently, over time, athletes could require a larger release of insulin with each dose of carbohydrate they consume.

Refilling the muscles quickly with glycogen after exertion is completely counterproductive, because low muscle glycogen is the state that raises insulin sensitivity. Restricting carbohydrate intake following exercise enhances insulin sensitivity for at least 48 hours. It also causes the body to burn more fat as fuel.

I suspect that many extreme athletes who overload on carbohydrates are setting themselves up for mitochondrial damage. They are flowing so much energy through oxidative metabolism pathways that their mitochondria release large amounts of free radicals. In time, these reactive oxygen species will damage the energy-producing mitochondria and reduce their output. I hope these athletes are not damaging their longevity or setting preconditions for cancer or mitochondrial decline. Free radicals (ROS) damage cellular DNA and are among the prime promoters of cancer.

It would be easier for athletes to sustain high calorific intake if they consumed more fat and less simple carbohydrate. This would reduce the load on the digestion process, too. But athletes fear that without eating massive amounts of carbs they will not replenish muscle glycogen quickly enough for the next training session. I don't know that the evidence fully supports that point of view. Nor does it follow that the carbs must be taken every day to bring muscle glycogen to optimal level. The literature is appallingly weak regarding diets for athletics. Nor is it clear what the rate of glycogen repletion is following a training session.

This much we *do* know: a low-carb diet leads to a reduction in athletic performance. That is the consensus view and has been shown in a long line of studies. However, none of these studies allowed a sufficient period of adaptation by the athlete to the diet. It takes weeks to adjust to a low-carbohydrate diet, and none of the studies allowed sufficient time for that. So, the question remains open.

On the other hand, the consequence of excessive carbohydrate consumption, even among active athletes, is not in question. It is eventually ruinous to health.

Contemporary hunter-gatherers have legendary endurance even though they eat little carbohydrate and certainly do not carbo-load before an event the way modern athletes do. Members of the Aché tribe of Paraguay expend 4,000 to 5,000 calories a day foraging, with meat and fat as their primary fuels (they also eat high-energy tubers that make a small contribution to their intake). The Inuit Eskimo eat a diet of fat and protein with almost no carbohydrate. They hunt and fish in cold, difficult terrain with ease. Native Americans relied on pemmican as their fuel, a mixture of meat, fat and berries. They could live for days on the energy, protein and antioxidants it supplied.

Stephen Phinney tested endurance and peak aerobic power of subjects after a six-week period of adaptation to a low-carbohydrate, moderate-protein, high-fat, very low-calorie diet, while making sure they had adequate sodium and potassium intake.

The average subject lost over twenty pounds in six weeks. Their peak aerobic power did not decline, a fact that suggests their muscles were not depleted of glycogen, which is their primary fuel. Endurance declined initially but then increased to a higher level than baseline at the end of six weeks. All this occurred on a diet that supplied fewer calories than the subjects expended.

In a second study, of bicycle racers, Phinney prepared the subjects for one week on their standard diet, in which 67 per cent of energy came from carbohydrate. This was followed by four weeks on the Inuit diet consisting of 83 per cent of energy as fat, 15 per cent as protein, and less than 3 per cent as carbohydrate. To maintain mineral balance during the adjustment period, the subjects were supplemented with 1g of potassium, 3g of sodium, 600mg of calcium, 300mg of magnesium and a standard multivitamin.

The cyclists noted a modest decline in energy during the first week of the Inuit diet, but after that their endurance returned to baseline. There was a decline in the first two weeks in sprint performance, due to declining muscle glycogen of 2 per cent. By the end of the study, though, maximum oxygen expenditure returned to baseline and endurance time had increased slightly. The subjects were using fat, not carbs, to fuel their activity. These studies have not been refuted and consistent results have been found in animal studies that show adequate glycogen repletion and endurance performance of rats on a high-fat diet.

I am not arguing in favour of a high-fat diet. The philosophy I am advocating is moderate fat. But I am pointing out that the research does not support the necessity of a high-carbohydrate diet unequivocally, and that the health hazards of high-carbohydrate intake and extreme exercise are real and serious.

When training ceases, the visceral adipose tissue (VAT) is no longer kept in check and begins to accumulate more fat. Sumo wrestlers are fat but have small VAT deposits because their intense training limits its mass. When the sport is over, the VAT gains size and begins to sabotage metabolism. Insulin sensitivity, therefore, declines as the VAT tissues secrete hormones and cytokines that promote insulin resistance and inflammation.

With the cessation of hard training, and the dietary habits developed over years of training, weight management can become a problem for the inactive or less active athlete. The brain is now resistant to the action of insulin thanks to years of high-carbohydrate abuse, and it lives on the edge of glucose starvation. The retired athlete will find that he or she 'needs' glucose or starch to avoid feeling edgy and tired. They will feel the need to return to old foods and eating habits, which are hard to resist: every dose of glucose that courses through the body triggers a burst of free radicals that damage the appetite-control cells of the brain.

All human brains are biased toward excess energy intake and low energy expenditure, as we discussed earlier. This is the 'lazy overeater' evolutionary adaptation. Consequently, many former athletes find it difficult not to overeat, and carbs are their primary vice. Most former professional athletes gain weight, and many develop diabetes.

seven
the competition within

It may be true that once you start to look for Darwinism you find it everywhere. But it is also undeniable that inside us, as outside, there exist fierce competitions for survival. Outside, there is the struggle over resources, and only the genes that best fit their environment survive. One bird's beak is just marginally better equipped to get at its food source, and his shorter-beaked neighbour exits the stage for good. Inside us, there are similar battles for dominance being fought. Every cell in the body is an individual. Even though each cell has the same DNA as every other cell, the DNA is expressed individually and the cell must capture nutrients and energy that other cells also seek. There are even good guys and bad guys, since the winner will often determine the state of our health. Here are three of the key contests going on inside you even as you read these words.

YOUR BRAIN VERSUS YOUR PANCREAS

Or, to be more precise, your brain versus insulin.

The following explanation is kind of tricky because it involves one of the complex hormonal cascades that characterise the metabolic process. So please pay close attention. At some point it will seem as though insulin is the bad guy in this battle, but it's not the hormone's fault. Blame the modern magic of food engineering.

Now then, let's start at the top. Your brain runs on just one type of fuel, glucose (in truth, the organ can also use two other substances, ketones and lactate, but glucose is the main course). The demand for it is almost constant, since your brain will die if it goes for more than five minutes without. When your brain needs a hit, it broadcasts the message: 'Send glucose.' Your liver responds first, releasing glucose it has saved for just this occasion into the bloodstream. Your muscles also contain some, which they contribute to the cause. Your fat cells, too, release energy they store.

And that would be enough to feed even an organ as greedy as the human brain – except that your pancreas has its own response to all that glucose in the bloodstream: it releases insulin. Now, some insulin is necessary at this point, because without it your tissues can't access glucose. But if too much insulin is released, it sets off a series of unfortunate events, and the modern diet may have conditioned your pancreas to do precisely that.

This means trouble because insulin has its own marching orders: 'Store glucose in muscle and fat.' Pull it right out of the bloodstream. Which is what happens to all that glucose you've just consumed, meaning not enough of it has reached your brain. Still starved and now truly impatient, the brain sends your body another message: *'Eat more!'* Your brain is worried because, as far as it knows, glucose is still a scarce nutrient, as it was 40,000 years ago (your brain has no idea what a typical supermarket aisle looks like). Even a little delay convinces your brain that death may be near.

You, of course, don't know why your brain seems so frantic. But you get the urgent message: *'Eat something!'* And off you run to the kitchen to do just that … but then your pancreas notices and releases even more insulin. This stores more fat, which causes your brain to demand another feeding. And so it goes, around and around. You can see how a person might become overweight.

Here's a good question: why would evolution, which has mostly been our salvation, have allowed such a faulty and dangerous system to prevail? Well, keep in mind that many millennia ago there were no foods capable of triggering a massive insulin release such as modern groceries do. The brain was well fed back then precisely because there was no grain, no simple carbs, no pizza or white bread to send your insulin soaring and then crashing. A typical kitchen today probably contains more glucose or glucose-elevating foods than our ancient ancestors saw in a lifetime.

The cereal section of the supermarket may be the most dangerous place your children can play.

Who should win? Your brain.

What to do about it? Your liver, muscles and fat are actually capable of supplying enough glucose to keep the brain fed without help from external sources, as you get from carbs. But in order for that mechanism to work properly, you need to lay off bread, baked goods, anything with sugar of any type, or grains such as corn, rice, etc. Give it a try.

YOUR MUSCLE VERSUS YOUR FAT

Most people have a simplistic understanding of the role of muscle and fat: muscle is there so our bodies can move and do things and look good, we believe, and fat is there ... why *is* fat there? We have the general sense that some of it is needed for 'padding' (as though you are a sofa), but beyond that we see it as a hindrance, a nuisance, a bad thing.

Both conceptions are wrong, of course.

Metabolically speaking, fat and muscle are highly active tissue. Fat (the kind we eat) is a form of nutrient, one of the three we require, the other two being protein and carbohydrate. Fat (the kind we store) is necessary as a supply of energy, which our brains and bodies draw on continually as the need arises. Fat wouldn't exist if there were no good reason for it to do so. But if we all ate as we did 100,000 years ago, we would store just enough of it to provide energy and not much more than that. In fact, the challenge would be to build up enough fat for times of food scarcity.

But, as we know by now, contemporary eating habits mislead our bodies into storing far more energy than we require. It's worth noting that if your body fat drops too low you will die, but there seems to be no upper limit on how obese a person can become and still go on living. Reports of 1,000-pound-plus individuals have become almost commonplace.

Fat crosses the line and becomes a health hazard when it constitutes too high a percentage of our total body weight. This question of body composition is central to good health. Essentially, you should be around 11 per cent fat if you are a male, 18 per cent if you are a female. Anything more than that and the fat begins to damage your health. It even becomes toxic.

It does that by releasing fatty acids that can be beneficial in healthy amounts, but harmful to excess. The amount that is secreted is proportional to the amount of body fat – the more overweight you are, the more harmful substances (including cholesterol and inflammatory cytokines) your fat releases. Cells in your body are continually dying and being replaced by new ones. That's nature at work. But when fat cells die, they release oxidised fatty acids; the oxidation is the result of your immune system attacking and inflaming the cell and its contents. Someone who is quite fat has a lot of fat cells and, therefore, a lot of cells dying and releasing their damaged contents to inflame other tissues of the body.

When fat stores become large, they also release hormones such as leptin, vascular growth factor, angiotensin and some proteins of the immune system. The inflammatory factors secreted by fat will age you prematurely, and they will make you resistant to insulin, prompting your body to produce too much of it for your own good. When that happens, your muscle and brain get less of the energy they need, since more of it goes into fat. That's the insidious thing about the process – fat wants to create more fat.

In addition to all that, abdominal fat physically intrudes into the space meant for your organs, muscles and blood vessels until it impedes them from doing their jobs properly. So you see, fat isn't merely sitting there, ugly but otherwise inert. It is an active hazard to your health.

Muscle, too, does more than is apparent to the casual observer. Of course, it has its structural and mechanical tasks to fulfil. But it's not a stretch to say that muscle actually acts as medicine.

Like fat, its role is also determined by the size of its presence – have enough muscle and it helps maintain overall good health; too little and you are in danger.

Muscle supplies amino acids so that your immune system can build killer cells. Muscle is the disposal site for glucose. The tissue burns energy continuously, meaning you can eat plenty and not gain weight.

Muscle is also a source of energy for your brain. It

contains amino acids the brain uses to make glucose, meaning you will need to consume less of it in food. Having plenty of muscle and keeping it sensitive with exercise will reduce the risk of you developing diabetes.

Finally, muscle gives you the physical capacity to do things, so you will do more. Muscle gives you ease of movement and loads your skeletal system so that you will not lose bone mass as you age.

Who should win? Muscle, of course.

What to do about it? Increase and maintain your muscle by challenging it on a regular basis, which means you need to move it against the stress of resistance. For most of us, that will require some time at the gym, lifting weights. You must also feed your muscle tissue with sufficient protein to fuel its growth. Rest it, too, so the muscle can restore itself.

GOOD STRESS VERSUS BAD STRESS

The very word 'stress' has taken on a solely negative connotation today, although without stress of any kind we would be unrecognisable even to ourselves. We have lived with it since day one – the universe was created by stress, and stress has played a part in every moment since. But there is good stress and there is bad, and while the latter is inescapable, we can minimise it while maximising the former.

Good stress is the physical kind. For our purposes, it is self-imposed activity – exercise of one kind or another. It could be lifting weights, it could be a bracing hour on the tennis court, or a sprint up a hill. It is acute, meaning it lasts for short, well-defined periods of time. Our endocrine systems experience physical activity as the same type of exertion hunter-gatherers felt as they went about their daily routine. We release certain hormones in response to acute stress – mainly adrenaline – that get us through the event quickly. Our ancient ancestors' emergencies also tended to be of the short-duration variety, the kind that the 'fight or flight' instinct was designed to handle.

Acute stress is good because it triggers an adaptive response that makes us resistant to all types of stress, not just the physical variety. Our antioxidant defences are strengthened when we exercise. Our hearts grow stronger and our blood vessels more flexible. Our nervous systems shift towards a more peaceful state.

But if the stress lasts longer, other hormones are released – cortisol, mostly, which is an essential hormone that keeps us alive, except when it is released in a chronic fashion. When that happens, and we are exposed to cortisol for too long, it actually costs us neurons in the brain, muscle and bone. Too much cortisol damages the nerves, too. And, unlike our ancient ancestors, we have lots of long-duration stresses, mostly of the emotional and psychological kind. Money woes. Unemployment worries. Bad marriages. Difficulties with health. The kinds of problems that fight or flight can't resolve. Punching your boss in the nose or fleeing your mortgage just aren't options.

And so the stress lasts forever. As with diet, evolution hasn't done such a great job of anticipating the way we live today.

Who should win? Acute stress of short duration.

What to do about it? Exercise. Move your body in a way that will bring you joy. Beyond that, you need to find a way to relieve or even dispel all the long-term emotional and psychological stresses that are doing you no good.

interlude
is the NED right for vegetarians?

The short answer is yes, so long as you get adequate vitamins, minerals, fats and protein, many of which are most readily available in meat and seafood. That's why we eat flesh, not just because it tastes so good.

But my question for you is this: *why* would you want to be a vegetarian? There are reasons for making that choice, I concede, but they have nothing to do with health, function or longevity. So unless you are doing so because of a wish to kill no animal, or because of the toll meat farming takes on the environment, I think you should reconsider.

Just a few millennia ago, it would have been impossible to survive as a vegetarian. Wild plants would have been an insufficient source of nourishment, especially for protein. The last vegetarian human precursors did not endure. Their brains could not develop because they failed to consume enough long-chain fatty acids and protein. They had to eat all day to stay nourished, and so they had large stomachs, small brains and little mobility. They were rather like gorillas – vegetarian primates.

Dental isotopes of Neanderthals show them to be just below the wolf in how carnivorous they were. They passed from the scene about 35,000 years ago, but Cro-Magnon (*Homo sapiens sapiens*) dentition reveals that they were only slightly less carnivorous than Neanderthals. And they are the predecessors to us all. In *Evolution and Nutrition*, Michael Crawford and David Marsh argue that the human brain requires more fatty acids (EPA and DHA in particular) than can be produced by consuming only plants.

Only in a world with a safe supply of food can one consider vegetarianism. But even then it is not an easy choice. A vegetarian diet forces excess reliance on high-carbohydrate, high-glycaemic foods. There is no other way to obtain adequate calories. Otherwise, you have to eat so frequently and so much that you can't be very active.

The few vegetarian students I knew at the University of California seemed to think a potato crisp was a vegetable. They ate so poorly I don't know how they made it through school. Babies raised without eating animal protein are at risk of underdeveloped nervous systems and small, poorly functioning brains. Many vegetarians I know have too little lean body mass, a stressed, puffy look, and are too fat – they're skinny fat. Countries like India, Iraq and Egypt, where vegetarianism is widely practised, are undergoing an explosion of type-2 diabetes. This is because they consume large amounts of rice and other carb-rich foods, destroying their metabolisms and sliding into insulin resistance, accelerated ageing and diabetes.

If you want to remain a vegetarian, I suggest that you take adequate B-complex and fat-soluble vitamins such as vitamin A. You will also benefit from taking a branched-chain amino acid complex, one with little or no sugar or near-sugars. And get adequate fats from olive and omega-3 oils. Our vegetables today are not as nutritious as when our ancestors consumed them. On the other hand, the meat we usually eat is far from what our ancestors enjoyed, containing too much saturated fat, trans fats, hormones and antibiotics.

I choose to derive the bulk of my food from plant and nut sources, but I still eat a lot of meat. Carnivores love the environment, too. In the US, free-range animals are raised on clean rangeland, which preserves open space. Vegetables and grains take up space and turn it into monocultures. Free-range cattle eat a variety of plants and insects and have less body fat or saturated fat. Game is excellent food.

eight
age like me

Caged lab animals live about three times longer than their wild relatives. We modern humans live about three times longer than our wild ancestors – 90 years versus about 31 for them.

But our prehistoric forebears remained healthy, fit, lean and strong right to the end. They retained their vitality into 'old' age because they were active and ate only natural foods (not that they had much choice in either regard).

We do not outlive them because we are superior in any way. It's just that we in developed countries don't have to worry about starvation, predation, infection, exposure, drought and all the other potentially fatal misfortunes that civilisation has tamed, if not eradicated.

Of course, we have plenty else to worry about. Inactivity, starchy foods and obesity lead to a loss of insulin sensitivity and a host of hormonal changes that accelerate the ageing process. We live longer than our ancestors did, but we spend a higher proportion of our lives in disability.

Your lean body mass makes a crucial difference between ageing well and badly. It's the 'active you' that is the engine which carries you through life. It's the store of protein on which your immune system relies to destroy pathogens. It's the measure of your organ mass and function.

If you were to lose 40 per cent of your lean body mass, you would be dead. AIDS, sepsis and other lethal diseases cause a wasting of lean body tissue. Sufferers die when their body mass declines by that 40 per cent.

Ageing, Western-style, is essentially the same type of condition played out over many years. So powerful a predictor of health status is the rate of loss of lean body mass that it seems to be part of the process of dying. Rapid protein wastage is a cause, not just an indicator, of death.

What we call 'normal' ageing is in reality the long-term effect of sedentary living combined with carbohydrate abuse. It's the accumulation of damage from too little exertion and too much insulin. After they enter their thirties, adults lose about 5 per cent of their lean body mass per decade. Most of the muscle they lose is fast-twitch fibre, for they no longer challenge their bodies sufficiently. They settle into the slow-twitch region and their most important muscle fibres atrophy. Because the elderly infirm do not and cannot stress their skeletons, they lose bone density. They become vulnerable to falls, since their muscles are not strong enough or quick enough to keep them upright.

Centenarians tend to have low fasting insulin and are strong. They are not fat. I love the story about the woman who died at the age of 115 after falling off a ladder. She must have been strong. She probably had very low insulin because she was thin enough to climb high enough to sustain a fatal fall. Low insulin with low fat is a self-reinforcing feedback loop; each fosters the other. Centenarians have evidently reached a metabolic state that turns down the ageing cascade. Insulin and physical strength are excellent predictors of expected life span past the age of 35, and become more important with each advancing year. Leg and grip strength are also strongly related to mortality.

Finally, inflammation plays an important role in determining how well or badly you age. Inflammation is a protective response of cells to damage, irritants or pathogens. It is intended to remove the injury and initiate the healing process. But persistent immune-system attacks on damaged sites harm the cells nearby. Prolonged or chronic inflammation results in repeated or prolonged injury.

As we saw in Chapter 1, your level of C-reactive protein, normally tested in a metabolic panel, is one reliable measure of inflammation. High levels are predictive of atherosclerosis and heart disease. A great deal of inflammation is a function of bad diet and insufficient activity.

If you know how strong someone is, what their insulin level is and how inflamed they are, you know quite a lot about how long they can expect to live. You can also predict how long that person will be free of chronic disease, and how much time (if any) they will spend in a nursing home. The occupants of nursing homes typically have elevated insulin, low strength and high levels of inflammation. They age badly. We can all do better.

*

Life is an event-counting process, and some events count more than others. Injuries, financial or emotional difficulties, deaths of loved ones: they all weigh heavily. So the first steps to ensure a healthy old age need to be taken while you are still young: get a good education, save your money and don't take unnecessary risks. (I won't bother giving you the best longevity-related advice of all: be born with good genes.)

Some debilitating life events are food-related, such as the number of insulin or glucose spikes hitting the body and brain throughout the years. Each one lessens insulin sensitivity and kills neurons. Cells are damaged, and they can take only so much of that before they commit the equivalent of cell suicide – they execute their built-in death program for the sake of their neighbouring cells and the survival of the organism itself.

Many of the aged are poorly nourished. They have little interest in cooking or appetite and do not prepare enough fresh, nutritious meals. As a result, they lack key vitamins and, more seriously, protein. They are often unable to retain muscle mass, which encourages them to overeat – their brains sense the lack of protein and seek to obtain it from food. Because their diets typically lack nutritious foods, this means they just eat *more* bad foods. The result is too much energy intake, too little actual nutrition.

Beyond getting more protein, the aged should focus on eating vegetables and fruits to reduce the acidity of their bodies. Ageing seems to advance the body towards a more acidic state, which increases the damage done by free radicals and also promotes the loss of skeletal mass.

Fortunately, it is simple to avoid the highly acidic state that seems to go with ageing. Cutting all grains from your diet is one way. Grains and foods made from grains are acidic. Vegetables and fruits are alkaline and tend to neutralise the acids produced from grains or doing exercise (unfortunately, exercising does promote the acidic state as a side effect). Secondly, I think it is wise to take a potassium bicarbonate supplement to neutralise acid (it has another benefit that we will come to later).

What you *don't* eat also counts a lot. I hesitate to suggest to older readers that they eat less, since that can turn into its own problem. But current research in ageing and life extension focuses on the connection between nutrient availability and gene expression, pointing to the value of briefly going without eating so as to turn on genes that slow the rate at which you age.

As discussed in the section on intermittent fasting, some people try to extend human life through chronic calorie restriction (CR). People who practise CR limit their intake to as little as 900 to 1,000 calories daily, meaning they live in a state of constant semi-starvation. Those who can tolerate this perpetual misery seem to show good biomarkers in tests, but they lose a good deal of muscle mass as the body adjusts its composition to their energy intake. They are, on the whole, less muscular and a bit fattier than they would be were they to eat more, because they alter their body composition to maintain the constant energy needs of the brain and metabolically active tissues.

However, other research now seems to point the finger at glucose rather than total calorie intake as the ageing culprit. If this proves to be true, then the people who practise calorie restriction may be starving themselves unnecessarily. Instead, they should simply cut their intake of glucose. It would certainly be a lot easier to live with than starvation. This is why glucose restriction rather than calorie restriction is one of the pillars of the New Evolution Diet.

Glucose restriction is also beneficial to mitochondrial function. The mitochondria are the energy furnaces inside our cells that process glucose and fat to produce ATP, the universal fuel within the body. The number of the mitochondria and how well they function determine the amount of energy available to the cell. Mitochondrial DNA is affected by excess levels of blood glucose. Even just a few days of exposure to high glucose may result in the accumulation of oxidised proteins and reduced expression of mitochondrial DNA. On the other hand, glucose restriction improves DNA repair.

Here's why it works. Our genes have their own priorities, number one being their own propagation. They have no particular feelings about whether we as human beings survive; they are in it for themselves. They don't keep track of our years, but they do receive information about us from the nutrients they receive, and they base their actions on what they learn. If they get plenty of glucose from carbo-hydrates in our diet, they intuit that there is abundant energy out there, since glucose was a scarce nutrient 40,000 years ago. Based on that message, they feel confident that the environment can sustain lots of our offspring. And so our genes feel less pressure to repair themselves.

Low glucose sends the opposite message: your genes can't rely on your reproductive prowess, and so they need to maintain their own health. That's precisely the message we want to send, even if to do so we have to trick our genes by cutting out carbs.

We can also send that message by burning fat instead of glucose. When bacteria are fed glycerol (a form of fat), they live as long as they do when they are denied calories through chronic caloric restriction. It appears that when the body has only fat to burn instead of glucose, it is a signal to genes that nutrition is scarce, so they must keep themselves in good repair.

*

A lean, muscular body promotes low insulin levels. I am ageing at a slow rate in part because my insulin is low. Low body fat also promotes low blood fats, most of which come from a person's own abdominal fat rather than from diet. But it is body composition, not just body fat, that is the issue; you must have the right balance of muscle to fat to promote the hormone drives that keep you young and your brain well balanced and nourished.

Your muscle is also part of your immune system. It functions as a reservoir of protein to proliferate killer cells when they are needed in your body's defence.

Exercise even improves the age-related benefits of calorie restriction. Exercised rats on a restricted diet live 10 per cent longer than their non-exercised counterparts. This seems to come from the former's enhanced ability to mobilise stress responses. Exercise in CR rats actually reduces free-radical generation, which is induced by exercise.

Intermittent, intense and brief workouts build muscle mass that burns energy continuously. They promote hormone drives that keep you young. They switch the body's metabolic pathways so that energy goes to muscle and organ mass, not to fat. The intensity of the exercise is the key to reaching the fast-twitch fibres of the muscles, which are in turn a key to staying young. Retaining your metabolic headroom through intense, brief and variable training promotes maintenance of lean body mass, organ and brain – you will stay younger and smarter than joggers, who actually lose those vital three kinds of tissue as they run.

If there is a fountain of youth to be found at the gym, it is strength training. Weight lifting silences or reduces the expression of at least thirty genes that promote ageing. It produces an acute use of energy restriction and, therefore, mimics some of the effect of calorie restriction. Individuals as old as 90 respond well to weight training and can double their strength within a few months. Most of the benefits of exercise can be attained in one brief (no more than fifteen minutes), safe and somewhat intense session of strength training per week. I would suggest two, even briefer, sessions weekly so that insulin sensitivity and sleep are enhanced by your twice-weekly exertions.

*

Ageing is a process of accumulated damage, much of which comes from oxygen, meaning internal rust. We've discussed this elsewhere in the book: we need oxygen to live, but it is a double-edged sword, for it also gradually kills us. Oxygenation fosters harmful free radicals (ROS), which attack healthy cells by stealing their electrons and promoting inflammation and cell death.

A diet high in antioxidants, from either plant-based foods or supplements, decreases the oxygenation and, theoretically, ageing. In addition, a low-glucose diet suppresses free radicals. It also limits the formation of glucose protein molecules, glycosylated protein or advanced glycation end-products, which cause linking of cells and tissues. This linking is bad for you because when your body combines ROS and sugar, it forms a glue that attaches proteins to one another and makes body tissues stiff and brittle.

Our grain-based diet makes us acidic, and acidification only increases as cells age. The more acid we are, the more inflamed we become. In turn, inflammation and obesity promote insulin resistance, which leads to more insulin, and the feedback loop becomes self-reinforcing.

My diet eliminates the grains, beans and legumes, and milk that cause acidification and offers the plant polyphenols and other compounds that reduce inflammation.

In a later chapter, I discuss the dietary supplements I take to enhance my health, but the subject also deserves mention here.

A key effect of inflammation is the depletion of glutathione, one of the key antioxidants present in the supplements I take. It increases the permeability of tissues in the body, which in turn allows immune-system cells to heal inflamed tissue. As an additional countermeasure, it might be advisable to take 50 to 100mg of potassium bicarbonate. This will favourably alter the sodium–potassium ratio and reduce the acid state of the body. People who are suffering from ageing, which is a terminal metabolic disease, would also probably benefit from the use of branched-chain amino acids to supplement the amino acids they lack in their diet. Using these amino acids is likely to reduce the appetite for empty foods and increase the rate at which muscle and organ mass is synthesised (I will discuss this in the chapter on supplements).

Exercise, combined with adequate intake of protein, promotes protein synthesis and turnover in the body, which seems to be another form of renewal that promotes the health of the organism.

*

All in all, my own experience of ageing has been a good one. By the numbers I'm actually better off now than I was in my younger days. My insulin levels have gone down over the years, as I've adjusted my diet and begun intermittent fasting. My good cholesterol has risen and my bad cholesterol has fallen, alongside my triglycerides and blood glucose. My blood pressure is where it should be. My doctor tells me he's never seen a testosterone level as high as mine.

Back in 1995, when I was 58, I had a test of so-called biological age done at the Colgan Institute in California. As I scan the list of 'biomarkers of ageing' I see the following readings of biological ages: 29 for cholesterol, 30 for blood pressure, 34 for glucose, 19 for body fat, 22 for reaction speed, and 23 years for grip strength. My overall biological age at the time was shown to be 31. Even if you have some scepticism for ratings such as this (as I do), it does show that I have young blood, which is a good thing. Of course, I had a foundation of strength dating back to my youth, training hard in the gym and remaining active and health conscious ever since.

Adulthood was not without its challenges, naturally. One was a more or less constant inflammation. The other was chronic lower-back pain.

The inflammation was due in part to a lack of antioxidants in my diet. Some changes in my eating habits – increased fruits and vegetables, plus some antioxidant supplements – fixed that, to a degree.

I was tested for rheumatoid arthritis because I had been suffering with the connective-tissue form of arthritis. I think this was from swinging a heavy bat in my softball days, when I had been a real home run hitter, which left my wrist ligaments vulnerable to inflammation. I was also working out incorrectly, doing too many bodybuilder exercises and too many repetitions. Once I switched to my new style of workouts and began eating better and taking antioxidants, the problem began to resolve itself. Yet even then it never quite went away until I stopped drinking beer.

I loved beer, partly because I drink huge amounts of liquid. Back then I went through up to four beers a day. But I would notice that my face reddened when I drank, a sign of inflammation. This is a clear symptom that you are allergic to whatever it is you're consuming. The almost paradoxical thing is that inflammation prompts a stress response, which releases adrenaline, which in turn gives you a little bit of a high. It's just one more reason you become slightly addicted to things that are bad for you. I think this is why some people say they can never give up bread or pasta or pizza: the hormonal response to the inflammation caused by eating grains feels too good to stop.

The back pain was to be expected. I had injured my lower back while racing motorcycles, and my mother also had back and neck pain. It's especially common among those who had been as athletic as I was. From baseball I turned to academia, meaning I was spending too much time sitting at desks, reading and writing, another cause of back pain.

My solution was to stop doing all the static stretching exercises that had been recommended to cure my back pain. Instead, I focused on the abdominal brace stance, as I described in Chapter 3. This way of standing and carrying oneself caused me to focus on tilting the pelvis in the correct manner to restore the proper curve in the lower back, and to lift my chin and heart. When I worked out, I made sure to stretch the hamstrings, which also returns the pelvis to the correct position.

It all helped. When I was about 64, a year before I retired from UCI, I was in the most muscular and ripped state of my life at 208 pounds. One day I was rollerblading along the walk at Newport Beach, no shirt, just shorts and the skates. I rolled through a little opening between four young women walking alongside one another. As I passed them, one started panting and pretending to chase me. I loved it – she must have been about 17 and had no idea I was as old as her grandfather.

A few years later, playing softball, I hit an over-the-fence home run and later made a diving catch in the outfield. When I came up to bat next time, the catcher told the umpire to give me a saliva test for steroids and to check my age on my driving licence. In my last game in slow-pitch softball (I was 71 at the time) I hit three home runs over the fence and we still lost. No wonder I quit!

I would say that my health has steadily improved over the past three decades. I have none of the old aches and pains. And, having maintained my good health, I think I have acquired a kind of wisdom. It's a love of learning and a perspective that comes from having abundant energy. I truly feel fearless because, by now, I know I can handle whatever life throws at me.

I can say that because, just a few years back, a lot was thrown at me. My first wife, Bonnie, developed what is called systemic vasculitis. This is a terrible disease in which the autoimmune system attacks the small blood vessels, causing them to disintegrate and collapse. This causes the body's microcirculation to decline, failing to deliver oxygen and nutrients to the cells. She began to waste away, body and brain. Over the course of two years she was dying, slowly. My mother, who lived near us, was also in declining health then, and I had both to deal with.

During the last year of Bonnie's decline, I had almost no sleep. It is an odd thing about people who are dying; they sleep during the day because they fear the night. I think illness makes the mind retreat into more primitive regions, where the dark of night still equals danger. To cope with the strain of losing my lifelong companion, I deliberately ate less, episodically, in order to trigger my stress resistance. I dropped about 10 pounds, to a low, for me, of 195.

Bonnie's bravery still inspires me in sad moments when I think about her. She kept her great sense of humour almost to the end, until the fear took even that. She often told me that she was unhappy at the thought of dying before my mother did. She felt that a wife should always outlive her mother-in-law. Well, she made it. Bonnie died on 22 January 2006. My mother, Ella De Vany, passed away on 21 January.

I got through this difficult time thanks to the belief that I did not have the power to save my wife, nor did medicine. In fact, her disease was so rare there were no doctors capable of treating it. Out of this tragedy came my attitude that I have only one moment of power, which is now, and that I can determine not the outcome but only the probable path.

I had to find a new life that did not revolve around caring for my wife. I was still in terrific health and felt I could do anything I wanted. I briefly considered running barefoot through the condos and dating women of all ages. But I thought better of it. At 70 I did not want to raise another child, which could have come from an involvement with a young woman.

My neighbour at the time was a nurse. She stopped by to see me often as I sat in the hospital, waiting to visit Bonnie. Six months or so after Bonnie's death, that nurse's husband asked me if I wanted to meet a friend of theirs who also worked at the hospital. I'm glad I said yes, because she turned out to be the woman I would marry. Once I met her, I had no interest in dating any others. She was close to my age, trim and full of life and funny as all heck. Amazingly – because she is a phenomenal cook – she even allowed me to prepare the meals we shared in my empty house. We dated regularly and laughed a lot. I think I fell in love the third time I saw her.

We went to Italy together so I could ride motorcycles on the Isle of Elba, where I proposed to her on the beach. We've been married for almost three years now. Her health was good when we met, but her doctor had been alarmed at her less-than-stellar metabolic panel, and her blood pressure was high. All these issues quickly resolved themselves when she began to eat and exercise as I did. She even lost five dress sizes in a few months. Not a bad way to grow old together.

nine
supplements

Eating well is crucial, of course, but even that is not always enough. However, I find that dietary supplements seldom work. So I take very few, and the ones I do take have been refined over many years and are quite minimalistic and inexpensive. My only focus is on maintaining lean body mass, excellent insulin sensitivity, high immune function, good mood and turning down inflammation. I do think my supplements are partly responsible for the fact that I have not even had a cold in more than twenty-five years.

My two main supplements provide amino acids and antioxidants. These are critical for several reasons: they help maintain proper body composition, and can even control hunger. Good mood and high immune function are intimately connected to amino acids, too. I think females are more prone to depression than males because their intake of animal protein is too low to sustain adequate neurotransmitter synthesis. Serotonin (the so-called 'feel-good hormone') levels tend to be low in females and that is, in part, due to their low levels of amino acids.

Another important use of amino acids is to assist the immune system. Muscle and diet are the primary sources of amino acids for the immune system to draw upon when it must gear up to fight an infection.

Inflammation is a systemic problem that reduces insulin sensitivity and damages every tissue in the body. While the fruits and vegetables in my diet provide substantial amounts of antioxidants, I also take a sophisticated product that provides the master antioxidant, glutathione.

Here is what I take and why.

Vitamin D
1000 IU (25 micrograms) each day

I get outside in sunlight most days, exposing my arms, face and legs on the tennis court or just walking, meaning I get plenty of vitamin D the natural way. I may get out by the pool or in my back garden without a shirt for a few minutes, too. About an hour of full sunshine can supply you with all the vitamin D you need. But many people don't spend enough time outdoors, and so they should use supplements. Children are particularly vulnerable, especially kids who spend too much time indoors. Milk is not a good source of vitamin D and, in fact, most of the vitamin D is added after it is processed. (Besides, beyond the age of three, I believe children should not drink milk. It is highly allergenic and actually increases stomach acidity, which depletes minerals in the bones. Cow's milk has many problems, unless you're a calf.)

Omega-3 oils
Fish-oil capsules, 1000mg with each meal when I do not eat fish

I make sure to take it when I eat beef or pork, to offset the high saturated fat content. Or I take cod-liver oil with a meal now and then as a substitute for omega-3. But I also make a practice of skipping both of these now and then, because too much regularity is no good; variation is better. Refrigerate the fish oil after opening. I recommend that it have the 5-star rating, but am comfortable with the product I get at most health food stores or drug stores, even supermarkets.

Melatonin
3mg half an hour before bed

This helps to deepen sleep and improve antioxidants in the brain. Melatonin is a hormone secreted by the pineal gland that restores circadian rhythm and is also a powerful antioxidant to the brain. Loss of circadian rhythm and shallow sleep disturb the complexity of heart and brain dynamics and are precursors to the onset of disease. I do not take melatonin every night, just whenever I have coffee after noon or feel my brain is a bit too busy. Taking it every night might cause the natural release of melatonin by the pineal gland to lessen.

Branched-chain amino acids
5g per day

I take this with breakfast. If you're trying to gain muscle you should take 15g with each meal for a week, then go off it for a week, and then alternate until you reach a healthy body composition. Women, who typically eat less meat than men but usually need to put on muscle, should take 5 to 10g of branched-chain amino acids three times a day, with meals. Men trying to add lean muscle should take the full 15g three times a day at least until they attain proper body composition. But remember to always take a break from your supplements routine now and again. Variation is good. Once your body composition is good, amino acid supplements are not really needed but they are useful to maintain muscle mass, especially for someone who is older, and they are a healthy way to consume protein without having to ingest a lot of fat that is so often found in meat these days.

Antioxidants

Last, but perhaps most important, I take a potent antioxidant supplement to kill inflammation. I use a commercial product called Ultrathione Health Packs made by Antioxidant Programs Corporation. I have taken it for twenty-five years and have less grey hair now than then, and still have all my hair even though it was thinning when I started taking it (hair loss is caused by inflammation of the follicles). I take one packet with breakfast and one with dinner; each contains glutathione (which is the master antioxidant), vitamin C, vitamin E, folic acid, and vitamin Bs 1, 2, 3, 5, 6 and 12. I would not take any other available glutathione because it is digested in the stomach and may not reach the cells. Also, it may be metabolised into undesirable products that could actually promote inflammation, though this is unsettled.

ten
the last word

Because this book was written by an academic, you've had to make your way through a fair amount of arcane information to reach this point. As a reward for your perseverance, I have boiled the practical aspects all down to what can fit on a single post-it. You can even tear this out for future reference.

In order to live the NED lifestyle, you should:

1   Eat fresh vegetables, fruit, nuts, meat and fish.
    Stay clear of grain-based carbs and sugar.
    Avoid potatoes too. Watch the alcohol.
2   Skip a dinner every week.
3   Exercise with intensity. Lift weights, run
    sprints (but don't jog or run long distances),
    play a sport. Your workouts should be hard,
    but don't spend too much time at it. Two or
    three times a week at the gym, a half-hour
    each time, is plenty.

4 Remember, the goal is to eat and exercise as
   humans did roughly 40,000 years ago, before
   the advent of agriculture or labour-saving
   technology. Just don't overdo it. Be glad
   you're here now.
5 Give up the command-and-control approach
   to diet and fitness. Relax, enjoy the process,
   and let it happen.

afterword
By nassim nicHolas taleB

Before the essayist Bryan Appleyard made the connection in his *Sunday Times* profiles, few people had been able to see the fit between my ideas on probability, empiricism and extreme events ('Black Swans') and the diet and exercise – rather, lifestyle – views of Art De Vany. Yet they dovetail into each other.

The story is as follows. In 2001 I published *Fooled by Randomness*, a treatise on how we overexplain matters and do not quite understand the role randomness plays in life. A few months after its publication, I received a letter from Art. He wrote to me the magic words: 'I am using your book in my course on the economics of extreme events as I *despise* textbooks.' They were magic because I too despise textbooks (and most textbook writers) and tend to flee what I call 'serious mediocrity.' My book was meant to be aggressively playful, and few people noticed it consciously before Art, in spite of the sales numbers. So I knew that more mail would come from Art, but never expected that it would provide the nudge that eventually changed my life.

In another email Art asked me, 'Do you put kurtosis into your workout?' but I did not understand why it was necessary to do so. What is kurtosis? I believed that infrequent events had a dominant role in economic life – kurtosis is the statistical name for the degree these high-impact events play into a certain distribution of outcomes – so putting kurtosis into my workout meant, 'Do you have moments of extreme workout?' I did not, and did not realize the importance for a while.

A few facts that will follow explain that I had some of the ingredients of what I call an 'ecological', non-ludic way of living (avoiding what Art De Vany calls the gym equivalent of a laboratory rat approach to living an 'evolutionary' lifestyle). But I did not make an obvious connection.

a) **Lumpy work:** I believed that only bureaucrats and distinction fools made a distinction between work and play. The Greeks scorned what they called the *banausai* (artisans), the modern equivalent of salarypeople, as they believed that such work led to physical (and moral) degradation. To them (and other classical cultures), being involved in these routines led to muscle atrophy, and the avoidance of devotion to the life of the city led to moral decay. Accordingly, I fought with my nails to become self-employed, with no boss to prove anything to, and I spent time doing nothing, hanging around lazily, and worked with as high intensity as possible when work was necessary, for just a handful of hours per week. Unpleasant tasks (like meeting clients, talking to someone wearing a suit and tie, talking to finance people, listening to boring professors) needed to be dispatched as quickly as possible. So I shortened their duration and increased their intensity as far as I could. The trading life fits such a playful model as it resembles the ecology of nature and the life of a hunter: long periods of meditative inactivity, spent lounging and reading, followed by cascades of frantic and intense toil. Somehow the 'doing nothing' wasn't really so, as I am certain that ideas come to those who know how to protect their intuitions from the clutter of the disease called 'regular activity'. Little did I know that I missed connecting the dots as I stopped short of translating these ideas into a fitness regimen.

b) *Fitness*: I was then under the impression that I was fit, as I regularly rode my bicycle to the office, a hedge-fund-style operation, from the New York suburbs to the hills of Greenwich, Connecticut, for a total of 50 km (32 miles) per trip. Note that I said *regularly*, which, as we will see, *is a mistake* but I did not know it. I also ate *regularly*, three meals a day, which, we will see, is an even bigger mistake. And, the worst mistake, I attended a gym where I engaged in a predictably regular weight training 'routine'.

c) *Carbohydrate avoidance*: Furthermore I was then convinced, thanks to my father who was an MD/PhD oncologist with a polymathic bent as he published in many disciplines, including anthropology, of the need to avoid all carbs, except for fruits. To him, an ancestral diet did not include any other source of carbohydrates than some fruits and vegetables. But I made a mistake as I believed that we needed to eat with metronomic regularity.

My beliefs were as follows.

a) *Inseparabilities:* Just as there is this modern post-agricultural separation of work and play, you cannot separate nature from nurture, diet from work and exercise, job content from hobbies, textbook from reading for fun. But, under the influence of the rationalistic literature, I foolishly separated the 'cardio' from the 'strength' workout.

b) *Decision-making under complexity:* My entire body of work is based on the idea that we live in a complex system with hard-to-see causal links, and an intricate web of interdependence. The human body is 'opaque'; we need to rely on what had worked for a long time, hence evolved through the lengthy and merciless evolutionary test of trial and error, rather than produce our own theories deemed causal. Furthermore, there are non-linearities in dose-response: a little might be beneficial, more may harm. Such non-linearitites make empiricism secondary to tradition – tradition is the result of a long series of trials that are recorded in the beliefs and practices of a society that survives.

c) ***Wild randomness***. The consequence is that the randomness we observe in real life is rather more 'rugged', more uneven, more dependent on extreme outcomes, than the one we study in textbooks and imagine in our mental representations. The type of randomness I call Mandelbrotian (or fractal) power laws is a different paradigm (in which extreme events play a large role) which tracks reality much better than the 'bell curve' taught in schools.

d) ***Platonicity***. I also believed that we make the error of rationalism, of being blinded by 'what makes sense' in many fields deemed scientific, against empirical evidence – we don't like fuzziness and seek easy certainties. This leads to experts in many fields, including medicine, working with beliefs that are totally unempirical, without even knowing it. So I believed that we are suckers for 'regularities' and tend to fool ourselves into believing they exist where there is none.

e) ***Evidence-based science and working with the black box***. There are methodological consequences to the opacity of the human body – the 'black box'. The body cannot be divorced from its environment. Nature (and its logic) comes before statistics (it is a better statistician and far better biologist), but statistics come before biological theories. Biological explanations are narrow and causal, which works poorly in a complex system. Yet we tend to be overawed by their 'scientific' concreteness. As

Richard Rorty wrote about a similar problem: 'Sciences other than physics become 'more scientific' when they can replace functional descriptions of theoretical entities (e.g., 'gene') with structural descriptions (e.g., 'DNA molecule').'

I spent a few years reading neurobiology and papers discussing the neural correlates of decision-making, how the left brain does so and so, and which neurotransmitter does what, to little avail – when simple papers in empirical psychology devoid of a single biological statement showing the result of cohort experiments turned out to be vastly more predictive. How could biologists know less than statisticians? People tend to be overawed by the scientific appearance of biological theories, against our past record – explanations change all the time. It is biologists who promoted the idea of consuming carbohydrates as a source of fuel.

To give an example of the two different approaches: people used to claim as a rationalistic theory that muscles burn more calories than fat. Now the current biological interpretation is that muscles help with insulin sensitivity, so food intake does not lead to a rise of insulin in the blood. Tomorrow someone may claim some other hormone plays a role in causing the same effect. But an empiricist would just invoke the regularity that people with more muscle mass are less flabby at an even greater caloric intake, that our ancestors had more muscles than office inmates, and that's that.

THE MISSING FIVE MINUTES:
PUTTING THE KURTOSIS BACK

So, when in his email on 'kurtosis' Art asked me if I worked out in a way compatible with my views on extreme economics and complexity, I did not get the point; I did not realize that there was an obvious divorce between my ideas on randomness and my lifestyle. I was under the rationalistic belief that exercise was exercise, and that a good life needed regular exercise – and never thought of looking at the evidence-based papers: exercise improved all these nice laboratory metrics but it has not been shown to make people live longer. I was making two very severe mistakes: eating and working out steadily – which was not what nature built us to do, and I never looked at the empirical evidence.

Nor had I realised it right away. For I was punished when, hit with boredom in the back country of Greenwich, I moved the office back to New York City and decided to replace my bicycling with gym attendance. I attended the gym the same exact amount of time as I did bicycling, yet saw myself swelling, gaining close to 25 pounds of adipose tissue in three years. Then I realised the following: that I did not understand the application of *my own* ideas on complexity and randomness. The reason I was fit did not come from the hours of bicycling I did every week. The reason is that there were two or three gruelling hills that pushed my heartbeat to about 210 beats per minute – only perhaps five minutes of severe straining workout every ride.

But these five minutes were all that mattered. When I realised that fact everything came to me in a flash, with the usual shame at not having properly connected the dots. I needed to 'put kurtosis into my workout'. Then I started reading some of Art's materials and looking for what insights evidence-based papers could offer us. And I kept showing Art the pictures of the stronger and leaner body. Three years later, the improvement does not seem to stop.

There is a need for environmental randomness. So I failed in applying my ideas on Platonicity and had a representation of human life that relied on regularities and certainties. The human body is a machine fit for a certain set of random outcomes – so it needs randomness, not predictability. We have been built under a set number of variations coming from the environment, a variety of stressors – and now we are Platonifying ourselves by depriving our lives of these variations.

So I will discuss the following two points in sequence: a) the need to put randomness into our life; b) the need to put kurtosis into such randomness.

MATCHING THE RIGHT RANDOMNESS TO LIFE

A gym is to physical exercise what a chat room is to social life.

Here are the main sources of variations experienced by humans in an ancestral environment that I can think about now:

* **Thermal fluctuations**: cold, heat; add to that dryness, wetness, high variations in the level of humidity.
* **Energy expenditure**: some days and seasons require more work than others, with periods of overexertion followed by long stretches of rest. Art showed, backed by research, that regular jogging and marathon running degrade your health; sprinting and interval training improve it. Walking is not 'for exercise'; like sleep, it is a mysteriously effective activity that, as we will see, is necessary for humans to operate – and it needs to be done *slowly*. We need to look at it the way we look at yoga and meditation.
* **Energy intake**: bouts of hunger, fasting, followed by feast. Add to that episodes of thirst. I never have difficulty making people understand that a training workout that stresses the body is beneficial to them – the difficulty I've had is in making them understand that the same logic needs to apply to hunger and thirst. Hunger had to provide some benefits. We often hear the recommendations: eat three meals a day, drink eight glasses of water, don't overdo it – just without testing, based on some rationalistic interpretation of the human body. Yet evidence

confirms the evolutionary argument and shows
that intermittent fasting strengthens the
human body by boosting the immune system,
improving brain function and increasing insulin
sensitivity (or something like insulin we don't
know about as yet).

* **Sleep duration**: our sleep periods had to
experience some occasional variations.

* **Negative correlations amplifying energy
deficits**: what's more, there has to be a
negative correlation between energy intake
and energy expenditure. We work hard in
response to hunger; there is no natural,
ecological reason to work hard if we are well
fed. What's the point of doing so? Yet the
prevailing wisdom does not seem to be aware
of this elementary evolutionary logic. A
predator mammal does not eat breakfast to
hunt; it hunts in response to the need to get
breakfast. Yet I hear all these rationalistic
statements devoid of any evidence about the
need to eat a big breakfast before starting the
day. To see how such nonsense is widespread,
consider that, in a *New York Times* science
article, the journalist Tara Parker-Hope*
answers a reader's question, 'At what point

---

* *NYT*, Tara Parker-Hope, 2 July 2009, 1.29 p.m.

before exercise should we be eating?' She writes: 'I like it to be an hour before exercise. We're just talking about a fist-sized amount of food. That gives the body enough food to be available as an energy source but not so much that you'll have an upset stomach.' In such a representation, no doubt inspired by thermodynamics, you imagine your body like a car's petrol tank that you would need to fill up with fuel before you drive to your country house. (Incidentally this can provide an illustration of the difference between linear science and complexity; complexity theory would consider the interdependence between the engine and the fuel.) Evidence-based methods show that this nutritional dogma has not a bit of evidence going for it.

Art convinced me that we need to train our body to go hungry on occasion (or, at least, deprive it of carbs) while remaining active, in order to burn fatty acids. It works by shutting down these on-demand sources of calories. Indeed he once explained that if we don't train our body to burn fat we could die of hunger with plenty of adipose tissue around the waist. And research shows that people on a keto-genic (low carb) diet eventually operate, after the detox period, as effectively as others on a high pasta and orange juice diet. The human body is a complex information machine, not an engine. Exercise conveys information, and genes up-regulate and down-regulate in response to stimuli – so taking the information machine outside its normal, pre-agricultural habitat leads to the disruption of its equilibrium (or its various states of dynamic equilibria).

MY DE VANY EXERCISE

Fractality: There are some stressors our ancestors encountered once a decade, others once a year, others once a week, others once a day. Hence a workout and diet regimen needs to match what follows.

a) *No moderate exercise sessions*: Either too little, or too much, way beyond what I plan to do, and with no set schedule. Never have a clear plan of how long to stay at the gym. So I would randomly push myself, with output as power law distributed as possible. It is a matter of bandwidth. The range of fatigue from regular exercise does not reach all areas of the body. I now spend between five minutes and (very rarely) two hours at the gym, working out harder as I get more tired. I spend on occasion several weeks without any exercise. But my total time at the gym per month averages less than I did before the ecological regimen. And I have no routine, and do not count sets, with a preference for free weights/pull-ups/dips/push-ups. Sometimes I just do push-ups and avoid the 'moderate' number 60: I do either 10 or 350, then nothing for a long time.

b) *No yoga – just long, very long walks:* I am a flâneur and a thinker by profession, so my only regular activity in life is long walks, which I tend to take every day. I try to take aimless walks of between one and two hours a day, and up to five hours when I travel. I also walk on uneven surfaces, which seems to stretch my back. When I can, I walk on rocks. I believe that gym rats and cyclists do not do negative exercises which are necessary for spinal health. Our ancestors did not do yoga and no stretching; they walked as an expression of being.

c) *Occasional sprints.* As Art showed, sprinting is fun, playful – and short. You know it will be over in instants and are too occupied to look at a clock, as gym rats do, to see when it should be over.

d) *No purely aerobic exercise*: The separation is foolish and not empirical. Avoid listening to 'trainers'.

e) *Food intake*: No carbs that do not have a Biblical Hebrew or Doric Greek name (i.e., did not exist in the ancient Mediterranean): no oranges (only citrus), no bananas, no mangoes, etc. Apples and grapes were acidic in taste, bittersweet. Like Art, I eat nothing out of the box. No sugar, bread, pasta, etc. Avoid artificial sweeteners. Rationalistic fools may tell you that they lower the calories, but they are trapped in their non-complex, non-information-theoretic thermodynamics – you do not know what sensors the taste of sweetness activates, what it up-regulates, what it does to your mechanism of equilibrium-seeking. Arguments based on classical thermodynamics used by idiotic nutritionists do not take into account feedback loops. We have enough evidence of people gaining weight (and perhaps messing up their brain) with the regular use of these sweeteners.

Also I tend to eat on occasion very, very large meals, like Sunday feasts, and feel satisfied for days later.

f) ***Starvation*:** Work out while starving.

So good luck with the regimen. I've been on it for close to three years and my intellectual production keeps getting greater.

acknowledgements

A few key people and events do change your life. I owe much to my many and enthusiastic blog readers. They have taught me much and their success stories inspire me every day. I would not have written this book without their inspiration. Bryan Appleyard's article about me and 'the diet that really works' in the *The Times* was a turning point in the progression of this work. His 28-pound weight loss on the New Evolution Diet is his reward. Had Nassim Nicholas Taleb not introduced Bryan to me, this book might not exist. Thanks, Nassim, for creating this 'black swan' event, and thanks, Bryan, for so accurately and passionately capturing the essentials of my evolutionary approach. I deeply appreciate the enthusiasm and commitment of my publishers Ebury and Rodale to this revolutionary concept of the New Evolution Diet and Lifestyle. Miranda West of Ebury offered comments and useful advice at every turn and her support and enthusiasm for this book were infectious. I thank my agent, Richard Pine, for being such a reliable and supportive guide through the publication maze. My super editor, Bill Tonelli, crafted my academic writing into the highly accessible and graceful prose you see here on every page. Thanks, Bill, and my readers thank you.

bibliography

I have sketched out here some of the research that may deepen your understanding of the key ideas I put forth in the book. A complete bibliography is available on my website at www.arthurdevany.com.

THE ACT OF WILLPOWER COSTS ENERGY AND DEPLETES GLUCOSE

See Matthew T. Gailliot and Roy F. Baumeister, 'The Physiology of Willpower: Linking Blood Glucose to Self-Control', *Personality and Social Psychology Review*, 2007, 11; 303, and Zheng and Berthoud, 'Neural Systems Controlling the Drive to Eat: Mind Versus Metabolism', *Physiology*, 2008, 23 (2), 75–83.

FAT SECRETES HORMONES AND SIGNALLING MOLECULES THAT AFFECT INSULIN RESISTANCE, IMMUNITY AND INFLAMMATION

See Antuna-Puente *et al*, 'Adipokines: The Missing Link between Insulin Resistance and Obesity', *Diabetes and*

Metabolism, 2008, 34, 2–11, and Pietro A. Tataranni and Emilio Ortega, 'A Burning Question: Does an Adipokine-Induced Activation of the Immune System Mediate the Effect of Overnutrition on Type 2 Diabetes?' *Diabetes*, 2005, 54 (April), and Wellen and Hotamisligil, 'Inflammation, Stress, and Diabetes', *Journal of Clinical Investigation*, 2005, 115 (5), 1111–19. See also the positive effects of exercise on the hormones secreted by fat in J. Berggen, M. Hulver *et al*, 'Fat as an Endocrine Organ: Influence of Exercise', *Journal of Applied Physiology*, 2005, 99.

DOES GLUCOSE RESTRICTION OR CALORIE RESTRICTION INCREASE LONGEVITY?

A good deal of ageing research has focused on the insulin/IGF-1 pathway, implicating insulin as a key component of the ageing pathways. Since insulin is deeply involved in glucose metabolism and storage, this suggests that glucose may be an important signal of the ageing mechanisms. The insulin/IGF-1 pathway is ancient and exists in most organisms. When nutrients are abundant, the insulin/IGF-1 signalling (IIS) pathway promotes growth and energy storage but shortens life span; see Wang *et al*, 'JNK Extends Life Span and Limits Growth by Antagonizing Cellular and Organism-Wide Responses to Insulin Signaling', *Cell*, 2005, 121 (8 April 2005).

On how ancient this pathway is, see Barbieri *et al*, 'Insulin/IGF-I Signaling Pathway: an Evolutionarily Conserved Mechanism of Longevity from Yeast to

Humans', *American Journal of Physiology – Endocrinology and Metabolism*, 2003, 285, E1064–E10171.

Dramatic new results that directly implicate glucose in longevity is the study of S. Lee, C. Murphy and C. Kenyon, 'Glucose Shortens the Life Span of C. elegans by Down-regulating DAF-16/FOXO Activity and Aquaporin Gene Expression', *Cell Metabolism*, 2009, 10 (4 November), 379–91. This important article caused the researchers to drop sugars and simple starches from their diets immediately following their discovery, and is summarised in *Cell Press*, 2009 (5 November) and *Science Daily* in 'Spoonful Of Sugar Makes the Worms' Life Span Go Down'.

Following the Kenyon team's results for worms is another finding in humans that 'restricting consumption of glucose, the most common dietary sugar, can extend the life of healthy human-lung cells and speed the death of precancerous human-lung cells, reducing cancer's spread and growth rate', University of Alabama at Birmingham, 2009, (18 December). Calorie intake linked to cell life span and cancer development: *Science Daily*, retrieved 28 December 2009 from http://www.sciencedaily.com /releases/2009/ 12/091217183053.htm.

Further support for glucose restriction is in the remarkable finding that switching metabolism to glycolysis, of the sort stimulated by intense exercise, may induce the longevity effects of chronic caloric restriction in yeast and other organisms that share the same pathways activated by caloric restriction (humans share those pathways), reported in Wei *et al*, 'Tor1/Sch9-Regulated Carbon Source Substitution is as Effective as Calorie Restriction in Life Span Extension', *PLOS Genetics*, 2009, 5 (5), e1000467.

I find it very satisfying to have been applying both these ideas – glucose restriction and exhaustion of muscle glycogen – to my own life for over two decades, long before they were discovered in the lab.

The persisting alteration of gene expression following that holiday 'I'll just do it this one time' bingeing episode is described in E. Assam, and D. Brasacchio, 'Transient High Glucose Causes Persistent Epigenetic Changes and Altered Gene Expression during Subsequent Normo-glycemia', *Journal of Experimental Medicine*, 2008, 205, 9. This is the mechanism behind the metabolic memory that I had found in my first wife's blood sugars following a big bowl of spaghetti or an episode of low blood glucose.

Stress resistance through calorie restriction is discussed in Yu and Chung, 'Stress Resistance by Caloric Restriction for Longevity', *Annals of the New York Academy of Sciences*, 2001.

OXIDATION, OBESITY AND AGEING

See J. Ault and D. Lawrence, 'Glutathione Distribution in Normal and Oxidatively Stressed Cells', *Experimental Cell Research*, 2003, 285, 9–14; S. Furukawa, T. Fujita *et al*, 'Increased Oxidative Stress in Obesity and its Impact on Metabolic Syndrome', *Journal of Clinical Investigation*, 2004.

The relationship of inflammation to loss of muscle mass in ageing is reviewed in Solomon and Bouloux, 'Modifying Muscle Mass – the Endocrine Perspective', *Journal of Endocrinology*, 2006. Their abstract is almost pure drama: ageing is associated with inflammatory chronic conditions such as obesity, cardiovascular disease, insulin resistance and arthritis. Sarcopenia – muscle loss with ageing – is multifactorial, with contributing factors that may include loss of α-motor neuron input, changes in anabolic hormones, decreased intake of dietary protein and decline in physical activity. Research findings suggest that sarcopenia is a smouldering inflammatory state driven by cytokines and oxidative stress.

Oxidation (ROS damage) plays a large role in cell death because a large oxidative stress triggers the cell-death program, as shown by Skulachev and Longo, 'Aging as a Mitochondria-Mediated Atavistic Program: Can Aging be Switched Off?' *Annals of the New York Academy of Sciences*, 2005, 1057, 145–64.

REINTERPRETING ENERGY BALANCE AND THERMODYNAMICS

Weight gain is driven by elevated insulin; increased appetite and reduced movement are the results of weight gain, not its cause. See Robert Lustig, 'Childhood Obesity: Behavioral Aberration or Biochemical Drive? Reinterpreting the First Law of Thermodynamics', *Nature Clinical Practice Endocrinology and Metabolism*, 2006, 2 (8), 447–58, www.nature.com/clinicalpractice/endmet.

Weight loss shows similar effects that, at first glance, defy the first law of thermodynamics (weight gain or loss equals energy in minus energy out). But a deeper look at energy expenditure induced by protein versus carbohydrate shows that higher protein diets have a metabolic advantage, so one loses more weight on the higher protein diet. See Feinman and Fine, 'Nonequilibrium Thermodynamics and Energy Efficiency in Weight Loss Diets', *Theoretical Biology and Medical Modelling*, 2007.

I show that energy balance is stochastic and that an evolutionary stable energy strategy for our ancestors required that they eat on average more than they expend in energy; see Arthur De Vany, *Why We Get Fat* (2003), available at www.arthurdevany.com. I call this the 'lazy overeater' strategy in the text.

Not all calories are equal. Questioning that a calorie is really a calorie is becoming serious research, as in Manninen, 'Is a Calorie Really a Calorie?' Metabolic Advantage of Low-Carbohydrate Diets', *Journal of the International Society of Sports Nutrition*, 2004.

EXERCISE

Short-duration, high-intensity exercise improves insulin sensitivity, gene expression and muscle. See Barbraj, Vollard *et al*, 'Extremely Short Duration High Intensity Interval Training Substantially Improves Insulin Action in Young Healthy Males', Herriot-Watt University, Edinburgh, 2009, and Singh *et al*, 'Insulin-Like Growth Factor

I in Skeletal Muscle after Weight-Lifting Exercise in Frail Elders', *American Journal of Physiology – Endocrinology and Metabolism*, 1999.

Exercising with low carbohydrate stores in the muscles, something that is almost anathema to runners and body-builders, improves the genetic response to exercise. Low carbohydrate stores in muscle improve gene expression response to exercise: K. De Bock, W. Derave *et al*, 'Effect of Training in the Fasted State on Metabolic Responses During Exercise with Carbohydrate Intake', *Journal of Applied Physiology*, 2008, 104, 1045–55. Exercise releases lactate and growth hormone.

The metabolic effects of high or low intensity exercise are examined in N.E. Felsing, 'Effect of Low and High Intensity Exercise on Circulating Growth Hormone in Men', *Journal of Clinical Endocrinology & Metabolism*, 1992. High intensity exercise produces a better growth hormone response.

The safety of high intensity exercise is examined in Warburton *et al*, 'Effectiveness of High-Intensity Interval Training for the Rehabilitation of Patients with Coronary Artery Disease', *American Journal of Cardiology*, 2005, 95 (1 May 2005), 1–5.

The importance of growth hormone to the heart and other systems is illustrated in Khan *et al*, 'Growth Hormone, Insulin-like Growth Factor-1 and the Aging Cardiovascular System', *Cardiovascular Research*, 2002. High intensity weight lifting is the premier releaser of growth hormone.

An excellent book on high intensity, intermittent exercise is Doug McDuff and John Little, *Body by Science*, McGraw-Hill (2009).

ADEQUATE PROTEIN INTAKE IS ESSENTIAL

See Thalaker-Mercer *et al*, 'Inadequate Protein Intake Affects Skeletal Muscle Transcript Profiles in Older Humans', *Physiological Genomics*, 2007, 85, 1344–52. See also Porter *et al*, 'Aging of Human Muscle: Structure, Function and Adaptability', *Scandinavian Journal of Medicine & Science in Sports*, 1995; and Pilegaard *et al*, 'Substrate Availability and Transcriptional Regulation of Metabolic Genes in Human Skeletal Muscle …' *Metabolism*, 2005. And see M.J. Drummond, M. Miyazaki *et al*, 'Expression of Growth-Related Genes in Young and Old Human Skeletal Muscle Following an Acute Stimulation of Protein Synthesis', *Journal of Applied Physiology*, 2008.

Having a complete intake of amino acids is important for controlling the appetite because the brain senses the lack of any essential amino acid and promotes more food intake to secure the missing or deficient amino acid. Methionine is one of the most important amino acids as it is essential to the formation of all proteins. The article says 'Methionine occurs in naturally high levels in foods such as sesame seeds, Brazil nuts, wheat germ, fish and meats.' The NED is relatively low in calories and assures a balanced amino acid profile. According to research this combination may reduce ageing; see Wellcome Trust, 'Balancing Protein Intake, not Cutting

Calories, May be Key to Long Life', *Science Daily* (6 December 2009), retrieved 28 December 2009, from http://www.sciencedaily.com/releases/2009/12/091202131622.htm.

OBESITY, METABOLIC SYNDROME AND TESTOSTERONE

See Michael Zitzmann, 'Testosterone Deficiency, Insulin Resistance and the metabolic syndrome', *Nature Reviews Endocrinology*, 2009, 5, 673–81. On the effect of visceral fat on metabolism see E.W. Demerath, D. Reed *et al*, 'Visceral Adiposity and its Anatomical Distribution as Predictors of the Metabolic Syndrome and Cardiometabolic Risk Factor Levels', *American Journal of Clinical Nutrition*, 2008, 8, 1263–71.

BODY COMPOSITION AND AGEING

Research tells us that loss of muscle mass is associated with ageing and may even be what ageing really is. One review summarises the connection thus: sarcopenia is associated with a reduction in muscle mass and strength occurring with normal ageing, associated with a reduction in motor unit number and atrophy of muscle fibres, especially the type IIx fibres (the fastest fibres). The loss of muscle mass with ageing is clinically important because it leads to diminished strength and exercise capacity. See David Thomas, 'Loss of Skeletal Muscle Mass in Aging: Examining the Relationship of Starvation, Sarcopenia and Cachexia', *Clinical Nutrition*, 2007, 26, 389–99.

Exercise in a fasted state promotes autophagy and high protein turnover, which is a key factor in ageing, as shown in Tavernarakis and Driscoll, 'Caloric Restriction and Life Span: a Role for Protein Turnover?' *Mechanisms of Ageing and Development*, 2002, 125, 215–29.

It may be that the many benefits of calorie or glucose restriction involve the effect of body composition on ageing. Research shows that a lean body composition is protective against cancer and metabolic syndrome; see University of Alabama at Birmingham, 'Body Composition May Be Key Player in Controlling Cancer Risks', 3 January 2007, *Science Daily*, retrieved 28 December 2009 from http://www.sciencedaily.com/releases/2007/01/070102104108.htm.

OBESITY, METABOLIC SYNDROME AND BRAIN FUNCTION AND HEALTH

See Gómez-Pinilla, 'Brain Foods: the Effects of Nutrients on Brain Function', nature.com, 2008, and Kern *et al*, 'Role of Insulin in Alzheimer's Disease: Approaches Emerging from Basic Animal Research and Neurocognitive Studies in Humans', *Drug Development Research*, 2002, 56 (3), 511–25. Does carbohydrate help or impede brain function? See E.L. Gibson, 'Carbohydrates and Mental Function: Feeding or Impeding the Brain?' *Nutrition Bulletin*, 2007.

If you read only one article about bad food and brain function, read Robert Lustig, 'How Our Western Environment Starves Kids' Brains', *Pediatric Annals*, 2006, 35 (12).

STRESS

A wonderfully written, science-drenched but readable discussion of stress is Robert Sapolski's *Why Zebras Don't Get Ulcers*, third edition, Henry Holt & Company, New York (2004). How stress, inflammation and metabolism are intertwined is covered in Wellen and Hotamisligil, 'Inflammation, Stress, and Diabetes', *Journal of Clinical Investigation*, 2005, 115 (5), 1111–19 and M. Dallman, 'Minireview: Glucocorticoids–Food Intake, Abdominal Obesity, and Wealthy Nations in 2004', *Endocrinology*, 2004, 145, 2633–38.

The failure of feedback loops to control stress is shown in M.F. Dallman, S. F. Akana, *et al*, 'Stress, Feedback and Facilitation in the Hypothalamo-Pituitary-Adrenal Axis', *Journal of Neuroendocrinology*, 1992.

Exercise is good for the brain. See Cotman and Berchtold, 'Exercise: a Behavioral Intervention to Enhance Brain Health and Plasticity', *Trends in Neurosciences*, 2002. I do have a problem with them calling exercise an intervention, but I always feel better after and it is because of the way exercise or play releases brain neurotrophic factor (a kind of growth hormone for neurons).

AGEING

'Can you Really Extend Your Life', Chapter 8 of Robert Lawrence Kuhn, ed., *Closer to Truth: Challenging Conventional Wisdom*, McGraw-Hill (2000), contains the transcript of the segment of the show I appeared in where I questioned the progress in extending life in face of the declining health and increasing obesity of the world's population.

Is ageing really an evolved mechanism rather than just the accumulation of damage? I think the answer is yes. Starting with the mitochondria, those energy furnaces in our cells, one of my favourite scientists, Skulachev, takes this topic to new heights. See Skulachev and Longo, 'Aging as a Mitochondria-Mediated Atavistic Program: Can Aging be Switched Off?' *Annals of the New York Academy of Sciences*, 2005, 1057, 145–64.

Skulachev shows why he is one of my favourite researchers in this article on a genetically programmed death program; see Skulachev, 'The Programmed Death Phenomena, Aging, and the Samurai Law of Biology', *Experimental Gerontology*, 2001. My approach to health and ageing affects every one of the key death programs noted in the article in a way that seems to be favourable.

Strengthening the point that ageing *is* a loss of body composition that I made in regard to inflammation is R.N. Baumgartner, 'Body Composition in Healthy Aging', *Annals of the New York Academy of Sciences*, 2000.

Reactive oxygen species damage muscle and contribute to the loss of muscle with ageing, particularly those fast twitch fibres; see S. Fulle, F. Protasi, *et al*, 'The Contribution of Reactive Oxygen Species to Sarcopenia and Muscle Ageing', *Experimental Gerontology*, 2004.

To be lean and have high insulin sensitivity are keys to living long and well, as this review shows: Klöting and

Blüher, 'Extended Longevity and Insulin Signaling in Adipose Tissue', *Experimental Gerontology*, 2005.

DIET

The power of nutrition to shape evolution and the importance of fatty acids in human evolution are beautifully exposited in Michael Crawford and David Marsh, *Nutrition and Evolution*, Keats Publishing, New Canaan, CT (1995).

Consumption of marine-based foods in human evolution is discussed in N. Bicho and J. Haws, 'At the Land's End: Marine Resources and the Importance of Fluctuations in the Coastline in the Prehistoric Hunter-Gatherer Economy of Portugal', *Quaternary Science Reviews*, 2008, 27, 2166–75.

The effects of consuming a hunter-gather diet are superior to the benefits of the Mediterranean diet, as shown in L.A. Frassetto, M. Schloetter *et al*, 'Metabolic and Physiologic Improvements from Consuming a Paleolithic, Hunter-Gatherer Type Diet', *European Journal of Clinical Nutrition*, 2004.

A very low-carbohydrate diet profoundly alters fatty acid profile favourably and reduces inflammation. See Bibus *et al*, 'Comparison of Low Fat and Low Carbohydrate Diets on Circulating Fatty Acid Composition and Markers of Inflammation', *Lipids*, 2008, 43, 65–77.

A telling reassessment of the low-fat diet as a treatment for diabetes and obesity is to be found in Dahlqvist *et al*, 'Dietary Carbohydrate Restriction in Type 2 Diabetes

Mellitus and Metabolic Syndrome: Time for a Critical Appraisal', *Nutrition and Metabolism*, 2008, 5 (9), 1743-7075. In the article, experiments are summarised showing that carbohydrate-restricted diets are at least as effective for weight loss as low-fat diets and that substitution of fat for carbohydrate is generally beneficial for risk of cardio-vascular disease. These beneficial effects of carbohydrate restriction do not require weight loss. Finally, the point is reiterated that carbohydrate restriction improves all of the features of metabolic syndrome.

Carbohydrate restriction shifts fuel sources from glucose and fatty acids to fatty acids and ketones, and carbohydrate-restricted diets lead to appetite reduction, weight loss and improvement in markers of cardiovascular disease, as shown in Westman *et al*, 'Low-Carbohydrate Nutrition and Metabolism', *American Journal of Clinical Nutrition*, 2007; and Westman and Vernon, 'Has Carbohydrate-Restriction been Forgotten as a Treatment for Diabetes Mellitus? A Perspective on the ACCORD Study Design', *Nutrition and Metabolism*, 2008, 5 (10). See also Paddon-Jones *et al*, 'Protein, Weight Management, and Satiety', *American Journal of Clinical Nutrition*, 2008, 87 (suppl), 1558s–61s.

Low-carbohydrate diets are comparable to or better than traditional low-fat high-carbohydrate diets for weight-reduction improvement in the poor fatty acid control of diabetes and metabolic syndrome as well as control of blood pressure, post-meal blood glucose control and insulin level.

This is shown in Arora and McFarlane, 'The Case For Low Carbohydrate Diets in Diabetes Management', *Nutrition and Metabolism*, 2005, 2 (16).

An unusually long follow-up period for a diet study of 44 months on a low-carbohydrate diet showed steady improvement in body weight and glucose control, as reported in Nielsen and Joensson, 'Low-Carbohydrate Diet in type 2 Diabetes: Stable Improvement of Bodyweight and Glycemic Control during 44 Months Follow-up', *Nutrition and Metabolism*, 2008, 5 (14).

See also a stronger point defining metabolic syndrome as the *response* to carbohydrate in Volek and Feinman, 'Carbohydrate Restriction Improves the Features of Metabolic Syndrome; Metabolic Syndrome May be Defined by the Response to Carbohydrate Restriction', *Nutrition and Metabolism*, 2005, 2 (31), 1–17.

The role of insulin in food preference and weight is clarified in Velasquez-Mieyer and Cowan, 'Suppression of Insulin Secretion is Associated with Weight Loss and Altered Macronutrient Intake and Preference in a Subset of Obese Adults', *International Journal of Obesity and Related Metabolic Disorders*, 2003, 27 (3), 219–26.

Loren Cordain, *The Paleo Diet*, John Wiley & Sons, New York (2002), thoroughly explains the eating patterns of hunter-gatherers and shows how to adapt their foods to a modern diet.

Gary Taubes, *Good Calories, Bad Calories*, Alfred A. Knopf, New York (2008), is an excellent review of the diet literature and a challenge to the accepted view on weight control and disease.

COMPETITION WITHIN

One of the most original and important theories of internal competition is Peters *et al*, 'The Selfish Brain: Competition for Energy Resources', *Neuroscience and Biobehavioral Reviews*, 2004. This is almost straight economics, with the hormonal and neural actors all put into play to see.

Peters and his co-authors ingeniously apply selfish brain theory to the problem of obesity in Peters *et al*, 'Causes of Obesity: Looking Beyond the Hypothalamus', *Progress in Neurobiology*, 2007. I had stumbled upon the economic model, naturally since I am an economist, as we worked through my wife's diabetes. I had only a few hints of all the complex metabolic pathways involved at the time, yet we had the same strategy worked out.

The energy-on-demand concept that I utilised to shift our diet towards low-carbohydrate, low-glycaemic foods and rely more on internal sources of glucose for the brain is elegantly demonstrated in this important article by Magistretti *et al*: 'Energy on Demand: a Mechanism for Astrocyte-Neuron Metabolic Coupling', *Journal of Neuro-chemistry*, 2003.

Together the Peters and Magistretti articles, and the many that cite and expand their models, support the economic model of internal competition and co-operation in human metabolism and health. It is not so strange that an economist figured this out as it turns out to be an economic problem.

Fuels compete for utilisation inside the body and insulin resistance is a strategy the brain uses to protect its supply of glucose. A discussion of this competition and the importance of insulin resistance is to be found in Wang and Mariman, 'Insulin Resistance in an Energy-Centered Perspective', *Physiology and Behavior*, 2008, 94,198–205.

Go back up to the Skulachev articles under 'Ageing' to see how cell-death programs help in managing the competition within. The abstract from his Samurai law of biology reveals the need for a death program for damaged or rogue cells: 'Analysis of the programmed death phenomena from mitochondria (mitoptosis) to whole organisms (phenoptosis) clearly shows that suicide programs are inherent at various levels of organisation of living systems. Such programs perform very important functions, purifying:

1 cells of damaged or unwanted (for other reasons) organelles,
2 tissues from unwanted cells,
3 organisms from organs transiently appearing during ontogenesis, and
4 communities of organisms from unwanted individuals.

Brain and body compete for fuel and nutrients and, in the obese, the brain loses some of its essential supplies and parts of it shrink, as shown in Raji *et al*, 'Brain Structure and Obesity', *Human Brain Mapping*, 2009, published online.

COMPLEXITY, FRACTALS AND CHAOS

An early article linking complexity of the heartbeat to ageing that uses chaos theory and fractals to measure complexity is Pikkujamsa *et al*, 'Cardiac Interbeat Interval Dynamics From Childhood to Senescence: Comparison of Conventional and New Measures Based on Fractals and Chaos Theory', *Circulation*, 1999, 100, 393–9.

New models of human physiology and metabolism are expanding the idea of homeostasis to the wider, dynamic systems point of view. Recognition of the dynamic nature of regulatory processes challenges the prevailing view of homeostasis, which asserts that all healthy cells, tissues and organs maintain static or steady-state conditions in their internal environment. The new view, and the view I take in this book, is to rely on interacting, complex, dynamic notions of sustaining life far from equilibrium. Lewis Lipsitz points to this new way of looking at living systems in his 'Dynamics of Stability: The Physiologic Basis of Functional Health and Frailty', *Journal of Gerontology*, 2002, 57A (3), B115–B125.

A survey of the applications of fractal dynamics to disease and physiology is Goldberger *et al*, 'Fractal Dynamics in Physiology: Alterations with Disease and Aging', *Proceedings of the National Academy of Sciences*, 2002. They say that the non-linear regulatory systems are operating far from equilibrium, and that maintaining constancy is not the goal of physiological control.

Bruce West, *Where Medicine Went Wrong: Rediscovering the Path to Complexity*, World Scientific, Singapore (2006), shows the errors that result from considering the body to be a simple system, even multiple simple systems, and offers a way of replacing traditional physiology with a fractal physiology based on complexity.

SUPPLEMENTS

On the use of melatonin, see Kotler *et al*, 'Melatonin Increases Gene Expression for Antioxidant Enzymes in Rat Brain Cortex', *Journal of Pineal Research*, 1998.

glossary

Adrenalin: Medical name: epinephrine. Adrenalin is a hormone secreted by the sympathetic nervous system. It is also a so-called stress hormone that prepares the body for action. Neural transmission speeds are increased, attention is more focused, and the sympathetic nervous system in general is more activated. Adrenaline increases the heart rate, constricts the blood vessels so that blood flows more quickly through the body, and mobilizes glucose from muscle sources. It also increases tension and focus, and is one of the key hormones in placing weight on experience i.e. increasing the salience of events so that they are deeply recorded in memory, this is a natural role for a stress hormone like adrenaline because challenging experiences ought to be deeply encoded in memory.

Amino acids: The constituents of proteins, which make up the bulk of your body. There are just 20 amino acids in living things, though a few species have been found that use 21. Amino acids make up the structure and information of the genetic code – the letters of four amino acids, ACTG – comprise the alphabet of the genetic code. Our genetic machinery relies on amino acids. Your liver can make all the glucose your brain requires from amino acids in your diet or in your muscle. The immune system relies on amino acids to make killer cells. It is the most important ingredient in your diet for these and many other reasons. Fat comes next and carbohydrates finish last and are not even needed.

Body composition: The proportion of fat mass (adipose tissue) relative to lean body mass (muscle, bone, organ and nervous system). Humans are a bit fatter than other primates because our brains are so large and energy demanding. Primates living in the trees have abundant sources of fruit. The descent of pre-human primates from the trees to the savanna below made it a challenge to obtain enough energy in this relatively sparse environment. Insulin resistance and enlarged fat stores were necessary adaptations to the increased energy demands of foraging over the ground, covering increased distances to obtain food. Bipedalism (walking on two legs) and an enlarged brain were necessary adaptations to the patchy, scattered, and constantly varying sources of energy found on the savanna. We need our fat to keep our brain nourished, but fat can steal energy from the brain when there is too much of it. Poor body composition is ruinous.

Carbohydrates: A molecule composed of carbon, hydrogen, and oxygen. A non-essential nutrient the liver produces from amino acids or fat. Carbohydrates are used as energy to fuel metabolism and to store energy in the form of glycogen in animals or starch in plants. They function in the immune system and as structural elements such as cellulose in plants or chitin in insects. When the body is in a state of excess nutrition, it burns carbohydrate and stores fat.

'Clinically proven': In an advertisement the phrase means 'not true' or that they managed to find someone who lost weight while taking a mystery product, which proves nothing. A clinical trial is an experiment with patients who are likely not well; why else would they be in a clinic? Experiments can disprove (falsify) a hypothesis but cannot prove one. So, as a scientific statement, it is meaningless even though it tries to sound like science.

Complex carbohydrate: A distinction without a difference among carbohydrates first made by a Senate committee, not by scientists, that uncritically was carried over into government food pyramids. The USDA food pyramid is best called a pyramid of starch in my opinion. It has been called wishy-washy science and unfounded advice according to Professor Willet of Harvard University in his book *Eat, Drink, and Be Healthy*. A complex carbohydrate was defined by the Senate Committee to mean 'fruit, vegetable or grains' a distinction that at the time had little or no support in the research. The glycemic index and the insulin index were developed to measure the effect of carbohydrates on blood glucose or insulin to identify how complex they are. According to these indices, many 'complex carbohydrates' do not fit the notion that they have a low effect on insulin or glucose. There is no difference in a bowl of unsweetened corn flakes and a bowl of sugar. Most starches turn almost instantly into glucose inside the body. A russet potato has a glycemic index not far below sugar (85 versus 100). Ready-to-eat breakfast cereals are so heavily processed that the starches in them turn instantly into glucose. A starch is not a complex carbohydrate; starch is the storage form of sugar used by a plant. You don't need it unless you are a plant.

Cortisol: The primary human stress hormone, also referred to as cortisone. Cortisol rises in the morning to prepare us for the upcoming stress of the day's activities. It is secreted acutely, unless you are under continuous, chronic stress. It degrades muscle tissues and other tissues in the body to release amino acids that can be converted to glucose in the liver. The stress hormones act to maintain blood glucose levels; by inducing insulin resistance, causing muscle to resist the entry of glucose, sparing it for the brain. The lowest ranking chimp in a band shows what happens with chronic stress and elevated cortisol; the chimp loses clumps of matting hair, has shrunken muscle mass, a shrinking brain and a roll of fat around its tummy.

Fast twitch muscle fibers: The fast twitch muscle fibers are of several types: fast twitch type a, type b, and type x. The type b fiber is not found in humans (except in small muscles that do not move limbs), but is thought to be the wild type of fiber found in small animals. They are too fast to power human movement. The type a are called the oxidative/glycolytic fibers because they use oxygen and glycolysis to generate their rapid force production. The type x fibers run exclusively on anaerobic metabolism: they do not use oxygen to produce their force and rely on fermentation; they are probably the oldest form of muscle that moved living things before oxygen came onto the scene. A byproduct of their contraction is the production of lactate that the brain can use and which is also a primary fuel for the heart. Muscle can also recycle lactate as fuel. This makes sense in evolutionary terms because extreme force production uses maximal amounts of energy and glucose must be preserved for the brain during such a stressful time. Thus lactate production in the FT muscle fibers offsets the glucose requirements of the brain. The type FT a fibers are not as powerful and do not have as high a threshold for activation as the FT x type fibers.

Glucagon: A stress-related hormone that signals the liver to release its internal stores of glycogen. You can see that this is also preparation for the performance of some response or action. Glucose must be mobilized in order to fuel activity, and to provide adequate amounts of glucose to the brain during a period of time when the muscles are going to be activated and may compete with the brain for energy. Glucagon cannot do its job effectively when insulin is high.

Glucose: A carbohydrate that is used by the mitochondria to make energy. It is the primary, but not the only, fuel for the brain. Starch is just glucose in plant form. Table sugar is about half glucose and half fructose, another plant form of carbohydrate storage. Glucose is an effective, quick acting source of energy because it is highly reactive, meaning it interacts readily with oxygen and other molecules. That means it can promote free radical damage inside the body by reacting with oxygen and proteins to form misshaped, hardened (glycated) proteins in the blood vessels, eyes and connective tissues. Glucose triggers an immediate release of insulin; this 'fast insulin trigger' is likely a result of humans evolving in an environment where glucose was scarce. In a world of sweets and sugary soft drinks this quick storage response is activated often, too often, and sets off the cascade into insulin resistance and accelerated ageing by turning on the insulin/IGF-1 pathway often. You don't need it because your liver can make all the glucose your brain requires to remain active by converting fats or amino acids into glucose on demand.

Glycerol: A component of triglycerides or fats that forms the backbone to hold the glyceride bodies together to form triglycerides. Glycerol is, strictly speaking, designated as a structural carbohydrate. It is essential for the formation of fats and is released when the body metabolizes fat. It does not raise insulin so it does not activate the insulin pathway. Since it is a signal that fat is being oxidized it may be an indicator of nutritional shortage, which may explain why bacteria fed glycerol live longer than when they are fed glucose.

Glycogen: The storage form of glucose in mammals. It is stored primarily in the liver and muscle. Muscle glycogen is a local source of energy for muscle, probably there for a quick response to fuel the fast twitch muscles for intense, fight or flight response. It would take too long if muscle had to wait for its glucose to arrive from the liver. When the muscles are full of glycogen they resist further entry of glucose, a big deal because that means they become resistant to the action of insulin. That is why we are not in a big hurry to replenish our glycogen after exercise, a practice that is almost a fetish with many runners and athletes.

Growth hormone (GH or HGH): Growth hormone is secreted by the pituitary gland. It is the hormone that is primarily responsible for growth and repair. It acts as an energy mobilizer by preventing fatty acids in the blood stream from being esterified into adipose tissues. GH is an important hormone in the metabolism of fats. GH is released primarily during the deep alpha phase of sleep. Its release is very pulsated, which is to say that it is released in bursts. This seems to be an important property in its effectiveness. In fact, pulsing release is a key signature of all the hormones. Intense exercise releases GH abundantly.

Insulin: This is a key hormone that unlocks the cell membrane for the entry of nutrients. In order for glucose to enter the cell, there must be a signal at that insulin receptor on the surface of the cell. The cell responds by making the membrane permeable to the entry of glucose. Insulin opens the cell membrane of every type of cell in the body and thus is the key hormone for the storage of energy. In order to perform this function well you would expect that insulin would also silence the hormones that are responsible for mobilizing energy so that it maximizes its effect on nutrient storage. Thus, insulin has the capability of silencing or suppressing the power of signals from hormones like glucagon, leptin, growth hormone, and some other stress-related hormones such as adrenaline. Insulin is most effective when it is released in pulses. A dose of sugar or starch increases blood glucose, which raises insulin immediately. This is followed by a steep fall in glucose, which is followed by the release of stress hormones such as adrenalin (epinephrine) to restore glucose. The cycle is a shock to the body, leaving you tired and stressed.

Insulin resistance: At some point, the cell membrane becomes resistant to the action of insulin. This results primarily from a reduction in the number of insulin receptors on the surface of the cell. Or receptors may become less effective at permitting the entry of energy and other nutrients in the cell membrane. The loss of mitochondria in the receptor through oxidation and ageing may be a contributing factor in the development of resistance. The fluidity of the cell membrane is also crucial. If the cell membrane fatty acid composition becomes too saturated – filled with saturated fats or trans fatty acids - then it becomes less permeable and more resistant to the entry of nutrients. If the membrane fatty acids become oxidized, the membrane becomes resistant to the entry of nutrients. Insulin resistance is a defense the brain uses to protect its supply of glucose because it reduces the entry of glucose into tissues that compete for the brain's glucose. Insulin resistance was an adaptation that kept our ancestors alive back when glucose was a rare find; now it is killing us in novel ways.

Proteins: Complex chunks of amino acids connected together and twisted into important shapes. The shape of a protein and the way it folds and unfolds to expose parts of it is fundamental to its function. Proteins make muscle tissue, bone, teeth, and other structures. Proteins are the basic product of our genes. The dogma is that DNA makes RNA makes protein, which means that the information coded in the DNA is transcribed into messenger RNA which is then read in the ribosome to make protein. That is really all the genes do - make protein. Our genetic machinery cannot work without protein, which is probably the most important of the macronutrients – protein, carbohydrate, fat – for that reason alone. A protein is about 200 amino acids long; hence, the number of possible proteins is roughly 20^{200}! Just a portion of this vast number of possible proteins exist in living things and it took evolution a long time to sort out those capable of sustaining life. Most toxins are proteins, so it is clear that some proteins that do not sustain life have been put to defensive purposes by plants and poisonous snakes, spiders, and particularly castor beans, which contain one of the most deadly toxins.

index